AutPlay® Therapy Play and Social Skills Groups

AutPlay® Therapy Play and Social Skills Groups provides practitioners with a step-by-step guide for implementing a social skills group to help children and adolescents with autism improve on their play and social skills deficits in a fun and engaging way.

This unique 10-session group model incorporates the AutPlay Therapy approach focused on relational and behavioral methods. Group setup, protocol, and structured play therapy interventions are presented and explained for easy implementation by professionals. Also included are parent implemented interventions that allow parents and/or caregivers to become co-change agents in the group process and learn how to successfully implement AutPlay groups.

Any practitioner or professional who works with children and adolescents with autism spectrum disorder will find this resource to be a unique and valuable guide to effectively implementing social skills groups.

Robert Jason Grant, EdD, owns and operates the AutPlay Therapy clinic in southwest Missouri. He is the creator of AutPlay Therapy and author of several books, book chapters, and articles related to autism and play therapy. He is an international keynote speaker and trainer and spends his free time enjoying activities with his wife and son.

Tracy Turner-Bumberry, LPC, RPT-S, CAS, is a licensed professional counselor, a Registered Play Therapist Supervisor, a certified AutPlay therapist/trainer, and a certified autism specialist. She has over 20 years of experience working with children, adolescents, and young adults. She lives in Milledgeville, GA, with her husband, three rescue dogs, and bearded dragon.

AutPlay® Therapy Play and Social Skills Groups
A 10-Session Model

**Robert Jason Grant and
Tracy Turner-Bumberry**

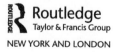

Routledge
Taylor & Francis Group

NEW YORK AND LONDON

First published 2021
by Routledge
52 Vanderbilt Avenue, New York, NY 10017

and by Routledge
2 Park Square, Milton Park, Abingdon, Oxon, OX14 4RN

Routledge is an imprint of the Taylor & Francis Group, an informa business

© 2021 Taylor & Francis

Library of Congress Cataloging-in-Publication Data
Title: AutPlay therapy play and social skills groups : a 10-session model /
  Robert Jason Grant, Tracy Turner-Bumberry.
Description: New York, NY : Routledge, 2021. | Includes bibliographical
  references and index.
Identifiers: LCCN 2020014289 (print) | LCCN 2020014290 (ebook) |
  ISBN 9780367410025 (hardback) | ISBN 9780367410018 (paperback) |
  ISBN 9780367810429 (ebook)
Subjects: MESH: Autism Spectrum Disorder—therapy | Play Therapy—
  methods | Psychotherapy, Group—methods | Social Skills | Child |
  Adolescent
Classification: LCC RJ505.P6 (print) | LCC RJ505.P6 (ebook) |
  NLM WS 350.8.P4 | DDC 618.92/891653—dc23
LC record available at https://lccn.loc.gov/2020014289
LC ebook record available at https://lccn.loc.gov/2020014290

ISBN: 978-0-367-41002-5 (hbk)
ISBN: 978-0-367-41001-8 (pbk)
ISBN: 978-0-367-81042-9 (ebk)

Typeset in Sabon
by Apex CoVantage, LLC

This book is dedicated to our families. Thank you for all your love and support. We could not have taken the time and energy to create this book without your understanding and encouragement.

Contents

Author Biographies   viii
Acknowledgments   ix
Foreword   x

Introduction   1

1   Autism Spectrum Disorder   5

2   Social Skills   16

3   AutPlay® Therapy and Social Skills   22

4   AutPlay® Therapy Play Groups and Social
    Skills Groups   29

5   AutPlay® Therapy Play Groups (10-Session Model)   43

6   AutPlay® Therapy Social Skills Groups
    (10-Session Model)   70

7   Additional Social Skills Interventions for Children
    and Adolescents   130

8   Conclusion   202

    Key Terms   204
    *Appendix: Step-by-Step Guide for
        Implementing AutPlay Groups*   208
    References   233
    Index   236

Author Biographies

Robert Jason Grant, EdD, owns and operates the AutPlay Therapy clinic in southwest Missouri. He specializes in working with children, adolescents, and families affected by autism spectrum disorder (ASD), ADHD, and other neurodevelopmental disorders. Dr. Grant is an international speaker and keynote presenter having presented for the American Counseling Association, Association for Play Therapy, American Mental Health Counselors Association, and the World Autism Congress. He is a multi-published author of several articles, book chapters, and books and is a founding board member for the non-profit organization Stars for Autism. He is a current board member for the Association for Play Therapy and is also a part-time instructor in the Play Therapy Certificate program at MidAmerica Nazarene University (MNU). Dr. Grant spends his free time enjoying activities with his wife and son.

Tracy Turner-Bumberry, LPC, RPT-S, CAS, is a licensed professional counselor, a Registered Play Therapist Supervisor, a certified AutPlay Therapist/Trainer and a certified autism specialist. She has over 20 years of experience working with children, adolescents, and young adults. Tracy owns and operates a private practice clinic in Georgia where she specializes in working with autism spectrum disorder (ASD) and ADHD. She also utilizes Carly, her certified therapy dog, in animal-assisted play therapy approaches. Tracy has presented and trained across the United States including presenting multiple times at the Association for Play Therapy Conference. She is also the author of several books and she enjoys living in Milledgeville, GA, with her husband, three rescue dogs, and bearded dragon.

Acknowledgments

Thank you to all the clients who have participated with me in play and social skills groups throughout the years. You have all taught me a great deal and helped with the creation of this book. I also want to thank my wife, Faith, and son, Nolan, who were always supportive and patient with my several writing weekends to finish this book.

—Dr. Robert Jason Grant

I would like to express my greatest gratitude to all of the people who have helped and supported me throughout my career. A special thanks to my husband, Michael, and daughter, Savannah, both of whom are constant sources of love and inspiration. Finally, a heartfelt appreciation to every client I've had the pleasure to work with, you all are some of the strongest people I know.

—Tracy Turner-Bumberry

Foreword

Several years ago, I reached out to Dr. Robert Jason Grant for help with my daughter. He was recommended to me by the doctor who had evaluated and diagnosed my daughter and also by several parents I had come to know in the autism community. Prior to meeting with him I previewed his web site and read about his therapeutic approach—AutPlay Therapy. I was impressed with the major tenets of the program, and today, I still consider Dr. Grant a most valuable resource in providing much-needed services for children and their families.

My story as a parent is similar to many other parents of children with autism spectrum disorder (ASD). I noticed subtle differences in my daughter as an infant that, with hindsight, proved to be precursors to the more obvious, atypical behaviors exhibited by the age of three. Early on, when the wide range of acceptable behaviors in free play, floating around to various learning centers of her choosing, and preference for parallel rather than reciprocal play were perfectly acceptable, my daughter was viewed as quirky, creative, and independent. Talking to the grocery store clerk and everyone else we passed at the store about how her "fishy died" elicited positive reactions and was cute at age three. But as she got older and most children her age had internalized social rules with little direct teaching, my daughter remained "quirky." She didn't seem to notice she was out-of-sync with the flow of ordinary activities such as morning and bedtime routines. She didn't appear to be socially isolated and was quite verbal, unlike the stereotypes of those with autism at the time. Instead, she injected herself into every situation with "bear hugs" and blunt comments.

By age nine, her social life had become exponentially more complicated—friend groups, sleepovers and keeping secrets were well beyond her skill set but in constant demand. Her mantra was, "If it is true, why can't I say it?" I struggled with how to explain these nebulous rules in ways she could understand. Instead of "quirky," she was now seen as "rude" and lacking in social skills. Middle school, as she described it, was "torture." The relative predictability of elementary school, with the quiet hallways and "keeping your hands to yourselves," was lost to busy, noisy hallways with slamming lockers. She developed a strict adherence to rules and routines. Typical kids figured out her differences and often used them to provoke her. Her individualized education program (IEP) became insufficient and she began questioning her very existence and lashing out at me for making her endure the situation every day. She became more frustrated and self-loathing as time went on and I was beginning to feel in over my head with helping her.

I read books and blogs, watched YouTube videos and went to presentations about how to help my daughter. I added a lot of tools to my autism parenting toolbox, which helped me get through the days with less confusion and conflict, but what I didn't realize at the time was that I needed a paradigm shift. I needed to see my daughter in a different light—from her perspective. What did the world look like to her? What did it feel like? How did she process her experiences that resulted in the behaviors she was exhibiting? I began asking her these questions and she was able to answer them with surprising self-awareness. She wanted friends, but her inability to grasp the rules of social engagement made it not worth it. How would she fare as an adult without these skills? Would she be lonely and isolated? Would she even care?

I had always believed wholeheartedly in the importance of socialization through public schooling, so I had never considered homeschooling. I believed in inclusion and wanted other children to also learn to interact with my daughter. The private schools in the area had fewer supports for her than the public schools. This was the point I reached out to Dr. Grant. He said there were very few (if any) real options for public or private schools that cater to the needs of students like my daughter. The only social group he led was for teen boys, primarily because so few girls were diagnosed with autism at the time. He gave sound advice and encouragement that helped us to relax and move forward with more confidence.

I decided to try homeschooling and it was one of the best decisions I have made for my daughter. We always say we "hit the reset" on her academics and socialization. We started with the parent-child bond and then slowly branched out again as she was ready. We also worked on an important project as an expression of this time together. With my daughter's input, I wrote the book, *The Alien Logs of Super Jewels*, a children's chapter book about my daughter's early experiences with the confusing world of social interactions. After writing the book, I immediately elicited the opinion of Dr. Grant as a reviewer.

After two years of homeschooling, we decided to help with the tremendous gap in school services and opened Infinity Academy, a school for middle and high school students like my daughter who need an alternative to traditional school settings. One of the first professionals I discussed this with was Dr. Grant. I knew he would know families who might be interested in the school, but more importantly, would have sound advice on setting up the social atmosphere for our students. He served on the board of the school and also led social group activities and parent trainings.

The positive impact of Dr. Grant's work is growing. He has published five books and he and Tracy Turner-Bumberry have conducted over a hundred AutPlay training workshops spanning four countries. I believe the reasons for this are two-fold: First, the demand for child-centered interventions is growing, especially as individuals with ASD's are getting more seats at the table in conversations about their needs. Secondly, at the heart of AutPlay is building relationships. Children invited into the world of AutPlay are seen as whole persons with all of the same basic needs and desires of any other child, and this includes close family bonds and social connection. Families are included in the therapy to promote these bonds and learn ways to integrate therapy methods during authentic social experiences in daily life. The result is a dramatic increase in the number of positive social interactions for the child. These positive interactions serve as reinforcement that drives the child to want *even more* interactions. I have seen these results in my own daughter and in the students I work with at my school. I am very grateful to Dr. Grant and Tracy Turner-Bumberry for writing this much needed book.

—Brenda Bradshaw, PhD, author, *The Alien Logs of Super Jewels* and *Autism—What Schools Are Missing: Voices for a New Path*

Introduction

Higashida (2014) stated that it is hard to believe anyone born as a human being really wants to be left alone and not have social contact. For people with autism, it is not having social contact that is the concern; it is the worry they may be causing trouble or frustration for others. This is why it is hard for those with autism to be around other people and they often end up being by themselves. The truth is that those with autism want to be around other people but because social situations rarely go well, they end up getting used to being alone. It's fairly understood that children with autism experience social functioning challenges and it's also fairly understood that despite the challenges, children with autism desire social connection. It is not about a lack of interest in a social life, it's about understanding how to navigate a social system that the neurotypical population learns and establishes with a mutual understanding that is not a naturalistic process for the individual with autism.

Most social skills develop without formal instruction in neurotypical individuals, starting very early in life. Most children acquire social skills as part of their typical daily experiences and developmental growth. Many people cannot recall how they learned to look at someone when they were talking or exactly when they first learned to get in the back of the line and wait instead of pushing to the front. But, somewhere these social functioning skills along with many others were learned and became part of their natural social navigation system. This is not the process for many individuals with autism. What seems logical, "normal," and even easy to understand does not always make sense to those with autism, and the social functioning rules are often challenging to learn and implement.

Unfortunately, many people expect a level of social functioning from children and if it is not present, expect them to quickly address the issue and begin to display the appropriate social skills. In addition, it is often expected once teaching children a specific social skill, they should have it mastered, without any additional practice or replication. When this does not occur (and it won't quickly or easily), the child is often penalized and sometimes labeled as resistant or defiant. For children with autism, social skill deficits are not going to develop because an adult tells them to do it, these social skills are not going to become an understood part of the child with autism's daily experience by punishing them when they do not display the expected social behavior. There is often a duality in need—helping the child with autism gain the necessary social skills to be successful in their interactions and endeavors while simultaneously educating those who work with children with autism to understand the unique complexities of social functioning and how to truly help develop these skills for those children in need.

Grandin (2008) said that she learned early in life that she had to learn social rules if she wanted to function in social situations. If she had to learn them, they had to be meaningful to her—they had to make sense in her own way of thinking and viewing the world. She developed a way to group social rules into four categories:

1. Really Bad Things—To maintain a civilized society, order must be maintained on some level. This would include things like not stealing, not injuring other people, and not committing murder.
2. Courtesy Rules—These rules are important because they help prevent anger and misunderstanding. Things such as general manners, saying please and thank you, and waiting your turn.
3. Illegal but not Bad—There are rules that can sometimes be broken depending on the circumstance. Things like slightly going beyond the speed limit.
4. Sins of the System—These are rules that must never be broken although they may seem to have no basis in logic. Typically, they are cultural, religious, or national rules. This may be dressing or not dressing a certain way, or not eating certain foods.

Children with autism often find the social-functioning world confusing, frustrating, and sometimes scary. There is a great need for them to develop the ability to categorize and understand social systems in a way that makes sense to them and enables them to navigate the social situations in which they are asked to participate. For children with autism to accomplish the social-related goals and experiences that are important to them, they must find meaning in social functioning. Koenig (2012) proposed that social competency does not develop in isolation from cognitive, emotional, and behavioral development. There is a continual interplay among these domains and competencies. When planning or implementing social skill interventions, the whole child must be considered, otherwise the interventions may not be fully effective resulting in gaps in the child's understanding and execution of newly learned skills.

Implementing any social skills intervention or approach requires the professional to see the whole child, not simply a child with particular social skill struggles or a child with autism. Understanding the diagnosis and common features associated with the diagnosis are essential for being a prepared professional but this should never replace or exclude the ability to see the fully developing child and respect the uniqueness of their abilities. There are several current approaches to working with children with autism: DIR/Floortime (Greenspan & Wieder, 2006), SCERTS (Prizant, Wetherby, Rubin, Laurent, & Rydell, 2006), Integrated Play Groups (Wolfberg, 1999), AutPlay Therapy (Grant, 2017), Theraplay (Booth & Jernberg, 2010), Replays (Levine & Chedd, 2006), and Autism Movement Therapy (Lara, 2016). Most established autism approaches include a focus on developing play and social skills but only a select few establish the therapeutic powers of play and specifically therapeutic relationship as core change agents in achieving social skill gains.

AutPlay play and social skills groups utilize play to help children gain valuable social skills. AutPlay groups present a relational based approach, which integrates elements of other established autism approaches, and can easily be combined with additional autism interventions. The child and parent participate in AutPlay groups, and specific focus is given to building the therapeutic relationship as well as building upon the child's natural interests. The self of the child is respected and his or her uniqueness is valued. Social skill development is built upon the child's strengths, and social skill interventions are designed to provide meaning for the child. This book outlines the process of implementing AutPlay play groups and AutPlay social skills groups and can be used as a guide for professionals who work with children who have autism or other developmental disorders. It serves as a resource for professionals to establish and implement play and social skills groups for children and adolescents. This book provides professionals with an adaptable protocol and tools necessary to create and lead groups to assist children in gaining social skills.

The AutPlay groups protocol describes how to start a group and highlights various group mechanics to follow that help ensure group success. The appendix provides several forms and documents that are used when beginning a group, and tracking documents that can help chart each child's success. These documents also help professionals collect valuable data when deciding on what type of group to implement. Further, several structured play activities and approaches for helping children and adolescents increase social skills are presented for professionals to use during group times.

Professionals can modify and adapt groups to fit their specific needs. Professionals are also capable of adding to or taking away from the basic concepts presented in this book. AutPlay play and social skills groups are flexible and adaptable. There are many successful ways to expose children and adolescents with autism to social situations where they can gain important social skills. Professionals can feel confident using this approach and integrating methods to meet the unique needs of a particular group. AutPlay groups assist children in gaining needed social skills by providing a supportive and playful structure to learn and grow. Professionals should strive to maintain a balance between the therapeutic powers of playful relationship and the evidence-based practice of social skill interventions. AutPlay groups support the integration of these components to create the most honoring and sustainable approach to social skill gain.

1 Autism Spectrum Disorder

The Autism Society of America (2019) described autism spectrum disorder (ASD) as a complex developmental disability with signs typically appearing during early childhood. ASD affects a person's ability to communicate and interact with others. ASD is defined by a certain set of behaviors and is a "spectrum condition" that affects individuals differently and to varying degrees. There is no known single cause of autism, but increased awareness and early diagnosis with intervention and access to appropriate services lead to significantly improved outcomes. Some of the behaviors associated with ASD include:

- Delayed learning of language.
- Difficulty making eye contact or holding a conversation.
- Difficulty with executive functioning, which relates to reasoning and planning.
- Narrow, intense interests.
- Obsessive behaviors.
- Rigid cognitive processing.

ASD is classified as a neurodevelopmental disorder that can be detected within the first three years of life. Typically, there are impairments in communication and social functioning. Those diagnosed with ASD can also have struggles with processing sensory information, deficits in play skills, motor impairments, repetitive behaviors, and challenges with change and unexpected occurrences.

The Centers for Disease Control and Prevention (2019), proposed that ASD is a developmental disability that can cause significant social, communication, and behavioral challenges. There is often nothing about how people with ASD look that sets them apart from other people, but people with ASD may communicate, interact, behave, and learn in ways that are different from most other people. The learning, thinking, and problem-solving abilities of people with ASD can range from severely challenged to gifted. Some people with ASD require a great deal of assistance in their daily lives; others need far less. A diagnosis of ASD now includes several conditions that used to be diagnosed separately: autistic disorder, pervasive developmental disorder not otherwise specified (PDD-NOS), and Asperger syndrome. These conditions are now all under the term autism spectrum disorder.

Children and adolescents with ASD may have some similar unifying problem areas, but the severity of their difficulty and the presence or absence of other features will vary, such as intellectual deficits, increased or decreased verbal output, and social strengths (Coplan, 2010). ASD is a spectrum disorder meaning there are many manifestations or ways a child or adolescent could be affected by autism. Siri and Lyons (2010) suggested that ASD is difficult to define; no two children have the same set of symptoms. Each child may broadly share common general manifestations but the triggers and causes for these manifestations may vary greatly from one child to another.

Children and adolescents with ASD are often misunderstood and mislabeled, especially when odd or unwanted behavior manifests. It is typical for children with ASD to struggle with behavioral issues. Behaviors can include shutting down behavior, refusing to participate, not following rules, avoidance, aggression, and executive functioning challenges, but are certainly not limited to just these behaviors. A variety of behavioral manifestations can accompany an autism diagnosis. Many of the behavior challenges that children with autism experience are due to emotional regulation problems, sensory challenges, and social functioning issues. Often children do not have the skill level to navigate situations successfully and the result is unwanted behavior.

When children with ASD begin to display unwanted behaviors, many adults working with them mislabel the behavior as purposeful or planned; behavior the child could control if they wanted. This is a dangerous mislabel as children with autism are often not in control when they are displaying unwanted behavior. In fact, it is a very out of control state for the child and usually a very frightening experience. Behavior struggles are to be expected when working with children and adolescents with ASD. It is critical that adults working with this population understand the dysregulation-driven behaviors children with ASD present, while also working to address the real issues creating the behavior rather than incorrectly labeling the child.

Academic and school related challenges are common issues with which children and adolescents struggle. The school environment could arguably be the most challenging environment for children with autism. The typical school environment presents social complexities, sensory experiences, rapidly changing processes, and adherence to a multitude of new people, activities, and routines. This presents a great challenge to children with ASD. Many children become dysregulated by the school environment and exhibit negative behavior, which at times, can manifest as large aggressive behaviors that produce additional problems. Some children are able to manage their way through a dysregulating school day and once they are home, explode into a meltdown. Many children with ASD will have an individualized education program (IEP) or a 504 plan which might provide accommodations to help the child navigate the school day more smoothly, but in reality, most schools struggle to meet the needs of children with autism and thus school challenges are a common occurrence.

A diagnosis of ASD can be thought of as a family diagnosis. Some children present in therapy with an isolated issue that primarily is impacting the child, but autism issues very much permeate throughout and affect the whole family. Many popular ASD approaches involve working with parents and other family members. Parents often participate in parent trainings to be better equipped to parent their child with autism. Siblings often participate in their own individual therapy to address the unique issues they may be experiencing having a sibling with autism. The impact of ASD changes the social and functional atmosphere of the family. Often times, the family's mindset, focus, process, and protocols revolve around the child with autism. Empowering and supporting families affected by ASD should be a developed component of any protocol designed to work with children affected by autism.

ASD is a Diagnostic and Statistical Manual 5th Edition (2014) diagnosis that is usually given after a thorough psychological evaluation; wherein, the evaluator measures the child or adolescent's behavior across a myriad of tests, assessments, and observations. The disorder is a spectrum disorder meaning the symptoms vary in intensity from severe to mild. Common terms used to describe the variance include low to high functioning, or severe to mild impairment. A synopsis of the manual's criteria for receiving an ASD diagnosis is presented in the following:

A. Persistent deficits in social communication and social interaction across multiple contexts, as manifested by the following, currently or in history:

  1. Deficits in social-emotional reciprocity, ranging, for example, from abnormal social approach and failure of normal back-and-forth conversation; to reduced sharing of interests, emotions, or affect; to failure to initiate or respond to social interactions.
  2. Deficits in nonverbal communicative behaviors used for social interaction, ranging, for example, from poorly integrated verbal and nonverbal communication; to abnormalities in eye contact and body language or deficits in understanding and use of gestures; to a total lack of facial expressions and nonverbal communication.
  3. Deficits in developing, maintaining, and understanding relationships, ranging, for example, from difficulties adjusting behavior

to suit various social contexts; to difficulties in sharing imaginative play or in making friends; to absence of interest in peers.

B. Restricted, repetitive patterns of behavior, interests, or activities, as manifested by at least two of the following, currently or by history:

1. Stereotyped or repetitive motor movements, use of objects, or speech (e.g., simple motor stereotypies, lining up toys or flipping objects, echolalia, idiosyncratic phrases).

2. Insistence on sameness, inflexible adherence to routines, or ritualized patterns of verbal or nonverbal behavior (e.g., extreme distress at small changes, difficulties with transitions, rigid thinking patterns, greeting rituals, need to take same route or eat same food every day).

3. Highly restricted, fixated interests that are abnormal in intensity or focus (e.g., strong attachment to or preoccupation with unusual objects, excessively circumscribed or perseverative interest).

4. Hyper- or hypo-reactivity to sensory input or unusual interests in sensory aspects of the environment (e.g., apparent indifference to pain/temperature, adverse response to specific sounds or textures, excessive smelling or touching of objects, visual fascination with lights or movement).

C. Symptoms must be present in the early developmental period (but may not become fully manifest until social demands exceed limited capacities or may be masked by learned strategies in later life).

D. Symptoms cause clinically significant impairment in social, occupational, or other important areas of current functioning.

E. These disturbances are not better explained by intellectual disability (intellectual developmental disorder) or global developmental delay. Intellectual disability and autism spectrum disorder frequently co-occur; to make comorbid diagnoses of autism spectrum disorder and intellectual disability, social communication should be below that expected for general developmental level.

The DSM 5 Three Levels of Support for ASD diagnosis:

Level 3: Requiring Very Substantial Support—Severe deficits in verbal and nonverbal social communication skills cause severe impairments in functioning, very limited initiation of social interactions, and minimal response to social overtures from others. For example, a person with few words of intelligible speech who rarely initiates interaction and, when he or she does, makes unusual approaches to meet needs only and responds to only very direct social approaches. There is inflexibility of behavior, extreme difficulty coping with change, or other restricted/repetitive behaviors markedly interfere with functioning in all spheres. Great distress/ difficulty changing focus or action.

Level 2: Requiring Substantial Support—Marked deficits in verbal and nonverbal social communication skills; social impairments apparent even with supports in place; limited initiation of social interactions; and reduced or abnormal responses to social overtures from others. For example, a person who speaks in simple sentences, whose interaction is limited to narrow special interests, and who has markedly odd nonverbal communication. There is inflexibility of behavior, difficulty coping with change, or other restricted/repetitive behaviors appear frequently enough to be obvious to the casual observer and interfere with functioning in a variety of contexts. Distress and/or difficulty changing focus or action.

Level 1: Requiring Support—Without supports in place, deficits in social communication cause noticeable impairments. Difficulty initiating social interactions and clear examples of atypical or unsuccessful responses to social overtures of others. May appear to have decreased interest in social interactions. For example, a person who can speak in full sentences and engages in communication but whose to-and-fro conversation with others fails, and whose attempts to make friends are odd and typically unsuccessful. Inflexibility of behavior causes significant interference with functioning in one or more contexts. Difficulty switching between activities. Problems of organization and planning hamper independence.

Beyond the criteria outlined to receive an ASD diagnosis, children and adolescents with autism typically have additional skill deficits and developmental issues. Splintered skill development is one manifestation that is common in children with developmental disorders. Splinter skills are abilities that are disconnected from their usual context or are very specific abilities that do not generalize to other capabilities. Because they are just a "splinter," or fraction, of a meaningful set of skills, splinter skills may not be particularly useful in real-world situations. Examples include the ability to memorize a bus schedule without understanding how to get to a bus station or buy a ticket. Another example is being able to memorize a multiplication table but not able to complete a multiplication question on a math test. Children with autism also display uneven development. A child with ASD may be at a developmental level far beyond their chronological age in one area of development and at the same time, far below their chronological age in another other of development. For example, a nine-year-old child with autism may have expressive language ability at an adult level (well beyond their chronological age) but have emotional regulation ability at a preschool aged level (well below their chronological age).

Due to the nature of splintered and uneven development, a child or adolescent with ASD will usually need an individual assessment to accurately identify his or her struggle areas, skill strengths, and skill deficits. Although it is understood that each child with have his or her unique manifestation regarding his or her ASD, there are some common deficit areas that tend to affect most individuals with ASD at varying levels. These common struggle areas include the following:

Communication skills—Children and adolescents with ASD will vary in their communication strengths and deficits. Most children with ASD will have some level of communication challenges. Some children will present as non-verbal, while others may possess a large vocabulary but lack ability to connect words verbally to their emotions.

Receptive language—Most children with ASD will have receptive language deficits. Many of these children may display average or above average ability in expressive language. There can be a large discrepancy between receptive and expressive language ability. Receptive language ability refers to the child's ability to take in or receive language. A child with receptive language deficits will likely not hear or process important pieces of information that are being communicated to him or her verbally.

Play skills—Children with ASD usually struggle in the areas of pretend or imaginary play and peer or group play. Regarding peer or group play, children and adolescents with ASD typically do desire to participate and interact with other peers in group play but lack the skills to interact successfully and find the experience to be too overwhelming. Thus, most attempts at peer interaction, especially with neurotypical peers, are not successful and may even create additional issues. Regarding pretend and imaginative play, children with ASD often lack the neurological process of understanding pretend, symbolism, and metaphor (Grant 2017).

Generalization ability—Many children with ASD will struggle with generalizing information. A child may learn a social skill in one context and have a difficult time generalizing the same basic skill to another context. There may be struggles with understanding nuance, learning through concepts, generalities, "it depends" situations, and pulling from an existing knowledge base to apply to new or unfamiliar scenarios. This is an important consideration when working to increase skill development for children and adolescents with ASD.

Rigid (literal) thinking—Children and adolescents with ASD may think in a rigid way. This means they may be very literal in their thinking, struggle with concepts, prefer more concrete thoughts, and find it difficult to consider alternatives or to accept when things are not how they expected or believed they should be. It can be difficult for children to think ahead and to guess what is going to happen next, which means they may become anxious or confused in some situations, especially new situations. Professionals and parents can assist children by establishing consistent and predictable routines while systematically introducing coping skills designed to help children process changes and manage unpredictable situations.

Processing speed—Research has shown children with ASD were found to have selective deficits in executive function. Executive dysfunction regarding attention, set shifting, planning, and processing speed have been reported in young children with ASD. Regarding executive function struggles, processing speed was found to be one of the weakest areas for children with ASD. Processing speed deficits present significant challenges for children in educational settings, home settings, or any setting where they are required to take in information and perform task completion.

Fear of making mistakes—Children and adolescents with ASD are prone to developing an almost pathological fear of failure, errors, or making a mistake. This fear may cause children to be resistant to trying new experiences or participating in treatment programs. Professionals and parents will want to reinforce a child's abilities and encourage self-confidence (Attwood & Garnett, 2013).

Regulation ability—A lack of social skills, play skills, ability to regulate emotions, and sensory processing challenges can all manifest a great deal of unrest and unwanted behavioral presentation for the child with ASD (Grant, 2017). This behavior manifestation is typically the result of the child or adolescent becoming too dysregulated. Most children with ASD will lack the ability to recognize when they are becoming dysregulated, lack the ability to regulate their system, and lack coping skills to implement when they are becoming dysregulated. Often, dysregulation behaviors can be misinterpreted as oppositional, defiant or purposeful behaviors.

Social functioning—Children and adolescents with ASD typically do desire to have friendships and interact with other peers, but simply lack the social ability and skills to interact successfully. Thus, most attempts at some type of interaction are met with rejection and anxiety for the child with ASD. Repeated attempts to engage socially, without possessing the appropriate social skills, can create a host of other issues including strong negative emotions that are difficult to regulate (Grant 2017). Social function deficits are arguably the most common issue with children and adolescents diagnosed with ASD regardless of where the child may be on the spectrum. Certainly, the level of social functioning deficits will vary but each child with ASD will manifest with some level of social challenge.

Perseveration—Refers to repeating or "getting stuck" carrying out a behavior (e.g., putting in and taking out a puzzle piece repeatedly), thought, or vocalization when it is no longer appropriate. Examples may include a child repeating a question several times within an hour or continuously manipulating sand with fingers for a long period of time. Typically, it is very difficult to move the child from the perseveration into a more adaptive activity.

Eye Gaze—Looking at the face of others to check and see what they are looking at and to signal interest in interacting. It is a nonverbal behavior used to convey or exchange information or express emotions without the use of words. Those who struggle with eye gaze may have difficulty realizing how someone is feeling or may not be seen as interested in participating in group activities.

Theory of Mind—The ability to attribute mental states (beliefs, intents, desires, pretending, knowledge) to oneself and others and to understand that others have beliefs, desires, and intentions that are different from one's own and this is okay. Children who struggle with theory of mind can become confused and upset when someone has a thought different from their own.

Joint Attention—The shared focus of two individuals on an object. It is achieved when one individual alerts another to an object by means of eye-gazing, pointing, or other verbal or non-verbal indication. An individual gazes at another individual, points to an object and then returns their gaze to the individual as they make a mutual connection.

Social Reciprocity—Social reciprocity is the back-and-forth flow of social interaction. The term reciprocity refers to how the behavior of one person influences and is influenced by the behavior of another person and vice versa.

Writing and other academic skills—Children with ASD tend to have an aversion to writing; they may prefer to listen to, watch, or do instead of writing (Attwood & Garnett, 2013). Many children with ASD prefer using a keyboard and seem to be more successful with keyboards vs writing. Writing should be approached with an awareness that children with ASD will need specific and realistic expectations and support. Other academic skills may also be affected and children with ASD may struggle in traditional school settings.

Self-reflection (introspection)—Self-reflection is processed differently by the brains of children and adolescents with ASD. Many children with ASD lack an inner voice or introspective ability and think in symbols and pictures rather than words. There is a challenge for these children to look within themselves, process strengths and weaknesses, then formulate a change/growth plan. Children who possess some introspection ability, will still have difficulty translating their visual thoughts into words. Professionals can help children gain self-reflective ability by utilizing visual learning tools to teach introspective concepts.

Self-advocacy—Milestones Autism Resources (2017) described self-advocacy as an individual's ability to effectively communicate, convey, negotiate or assert his or her own interests, desires, needs, and rights. It involves making informed decisions and taking responsibility for those decisions. Self-knowledge is the first step towards self-advocacy. An individual with ASD must know their strengths, needs, and interests before they can begin to advocate. Self-advocacy skills should be learned as early as possible and begins by understanding how to make personal choices, such as making choices about what to eat, how to spend one's free time, and what to do after graduating from high school. The Milestones Autism website lists several self-advocacy skills by age that children and adolescents with ASD should strive to accomplish (http://milestones.org/individuals-with-asd/self-advocacy/).

Grant (2018) put forth the following list regarding what to expect from children with ASD:

- Will likely have poor social skills and high levels of discomfort in social situations regardless of his or her level of functioning.
- Will likely poorly modulate his or her emotions.
- Will struggle with anxiety and high levels of dysregulation. Anxiety is typically the most challenging negative emotion for a child with ASD.
- Is usually experiencing some level of dysregulation, the question is how much? Many experiences can create dysregulation including poor regulation ability, a lack of social skills, new or unexpected situations, and sensory issues.
- Will produce most unwanted behavior episodes from a place of being dysregulated, which is typically not premeditated or controlled by the child and is often a very frightening experience for the child.
- Will have problems handling transitions, changes to his or her schedule or routine, and new people or experiences. Any spontaneous happening will likely produce anxiety and discomfort.
- May appear more or less capable than is the reality.
- May have small and large motor and coordination challenges.
- May experience a great deal of sensory processing issues in one or multiple areas regarding the eight senses (visual, auditory, tactile, gustatory, olfactory, vestibular, proprioception, introception). Sensory struggles can be challenging to identify and may involve environmental issues that seem benign to the professional.

- Will likely be a visual learner and prefer information presented in a visual format.
- Will usually be a concrete and literal thinker. He or she will likely do poorly with abstract or subjective thoughts and processes or information presented in this format.
- Most likely will struggle verbally to communicate what he or she is thinking or feeling especially when in a dysregulated state.
- Most likely will have challenges in receptive language ability even when his or her expressive language ability is high.
- Will likely be inconsistent in terms of skill ability presentation. He or she may accomplish something one day that seems very challenging and the next day is unable to accomplish something that seems much less difficult.
- May present with a great deal of hyperarousal or be the exact opposite and present with a great deal of hypoarousal.
- May be susceptible to being bullied at school and in peer situations.
- May be slow to respond to questions or tasks. He or she may need extra time to process what has been said or asked.
- Will likely experience school as the most demanding and dysregulating environment in which he or she participates.

When working with children and adolescents with ASD, it is critical for professionals to assess and conceptualize each individual child with ASD to fully understand how the ASD manifests for the particular child. Although there may be some commonalities, each child with ASD will present with his or her unique struggles, deficits, and strengths. Professionals are encouraged to develop a formal assessment procedure to help more accurately identify each child's skill strengths and skill deficits as well as any particulars a child might be experiencing due to his or her ASD. This process can be accomplished through parent completed inventories, professional observations, play time with the child, and obtaining background information from the child's parents. Grant (2017) developed a formal assessment process in AutPlay Therapy that involves conducting an observation of the child with the professional in a playroom, observing the parent with the child playing together, and having the parent complete several inventories to identify skill strengths and deficits in the areas of social functioning, emotional regulation, connection ability, and play skills.

Autism cannot be labeled as one thing, one "look," or one manifestation of symptoms. It is a vast and varied spectrum condition. The differences between two individuals with the same autism diagnosis can be many. The professional working with children and adolescents must remember the individuality of the diagnosis and strive to understand each child they are working with, especially in regard to their social skills and social functioning ability. It is this struggle in social functioning that may be the one unifying feature across the autism spectrum. Children will vary in what social skills are deficits versus strengths, how socially capable they are, and what particular social skills are difficult. Despite these differences, across the spectrum there will likely be social challenges. In this regard, understanding and addressing social skill deficits becomes a primary focus of clinical work with children and adolescents with autism.

2 Social Skills

Jamison & Schuttler (2017) observed that social competence is a complex set of skills that evolves over the course of human development. For those needing support in developing appropriate social skills, the importance of effective training programs sensitive to the unique needs of the individuals for which they are designed promotes the likelihood that skills will be learned and competence will be enhanced. Competence in social skills will then improve relationships and overall quality of life. Koenig (2012) asserted that children and adolescents with ASD have neurobiological abnormalities that make them less predisposed to engage in social interaction. Throughout development, children with ASD are less responsive to the social environment in general and do not benefit from the many implicit social learning experiences available from day-to-day experiences. Syriopoulou-Delli, Agaliotis, & Papaefstathiou (2018) stated that one of the core symptoms of autism spectrum disorder (ASD) is the deficit in social functioning. This deficit includes difficulties in initiating or joining social activities, difficulties in understanding others' viewpoints, engaging in inappropriate behaviors, lack of eye contact, distance from people, non-functional use of language, and a lack of communicative gestures.

The term "social skill" covers a wide range and variety of skills from simple to complex. Social skills can be anything from learning to take turns, to knowing when a situation is unsafe, to even giving a public speech. Social skills are interpersonal, specific behaviors that permit an individual to interact successfully with others in the environment. The extent to which an individual is considered to have adequate social skills is determined by others. This is especially true for children and adolescents with autism, as they may not be able to fully understand or recognize a social skill even after they have obtained it (Grant 2017).

A deficit in social functioning is a common symptom among all autism disorders. It is very likely that any child diagnosed with an ASD will need help in learning social skills. The negative outcomes associated with a lack of social skills can be many and serious. The inability to understand social functioning and possess social skills can create high levels of anxiety in children with autism and create problems in school and com-munity settings. Research has shown that these difficulties with social functioning are present even for the most cognitively able individuals on the spectrum (Reichow & Volkmar, 2010).

Early on, children with ASD demonstrate social skill deficits that differ-entiate them from their typical peers and classmates. In elementary school, they might have important relational problems such as difficulties initiat-ing and maintaining friendships with others (Kasari, 2016; Reichow & Volkmar, 2010). In high school, individuals with ASD might continue to show evidence of the same difficulties experienced in childhood, placing them at risk for rejection and victimization by their peer group. These problems could ultimately lead to social isolation, psychopathology, and poor academic achievement. Research also contends that individuals with ASD do not simply outgrow their social skills deficits; rather these difficulties might persist into their adult life and could continue to nega-tively affect their social functioning (D'Amico & Lalonde, 2017).

Social skills training for individuals with ASD may include a wide range of intervention strategies. These strategies include pivotal response train-ing, environmental modifications, social narratives, adult prompting, peer-mediated instruction and intervention, video modeling, self-monitoring, and incorporating typically developing peers in training (Murphy, Radley, & Helbig, 2018). Research supports social skills training as an evidence-based treatment for learning social skills. Further, research sup-ports peer groups as being effective in gaining social skills (Koenig, 2012; Ware, Ohrt, & Swank 2012; Grant, 2017). It is important to remember that social skills are learned skills. Every person learned the social skills they possess at some point in time. Whereas neurotypical children may learn social skills from observation, children with autism often need more direct instruction and replication. No matter where a child is at in terms of their current social functioning, they can learn social skills. Ashcroft, Del-loso, & Quinn (2013) proposed that successful social interaction requires effective social cognition. An important aspect of understating social interaction is determining what behaviors are expected in what environ-ments. Instead of teaching children that their behaviors are either appro-priate or inappropriate, children should be taught that their behaviors are either expected or unexpected in certain situations. It is important to teach children and adolescents the behaviors that are expected in a particular context and that the unexpected behaviors are the opposite.

Children and adolescents with ASD and related conditions will likely present with a variety of skill strengths and weaknesses. It is essential to properly assess each child individually to understand their social skill strengths and the deficits they need to improve upon. Working with the individual child on social skill improvement has benefits and certainly the child gains social skills through this modality. Addressing social skills through a group modality, especially one that is play-based with parent involvement, provides the opportunity for children to practice and gain social skills in a more natural, less stimulating environment. It also allows children the opportunity to practice social skills with peers. Social skill groups can also help children and adolescents recognize they are not the only person struggling with particular social skills, and these groups offer the prospect of connecting with peers and building friendships with other children and adolescents. There are many benefits to the group modality that cannot be replicated with individual social skill treatment approaches.

Barboa and Luck (2016) stated that appropriate social interactions are important for a happy and productive life. Forging friendships and having positive relationships with others is dependent on successful social interactions. Individuals with ASD may exhibit some or many social difficulties including:

- Difficulty making or maintaining eye contact.
- Inability to interpret facial expression or other gestures.
- Poor social or emotional connections.
- Little to no interest in what others are doing.
- Inability to see things from another's point of view.
- Difficulty understanding humor.
- Difficulty understanding slang and idioms.
- Have rigid, literal thinking patterns.
- Have extreme attachments to a toy or other non-toy object.
- May struggle with pretend and symbolic play.
- May reject or extremely crave physical contact from others.
- Display and repeat unusual motor actions.
- Struggle with changes to routine, or unexpected/unplanned situations.
- Exhibit high levels of anxiety in social situations.
- Resist situations that involve new people or places.
- Have difficulty with "small talk."
- Struggle with entering a conversation, staying in a conversation, and exiting a conversation.
- Struggle with asking for help and asking questions.
- Difficulty understanding friendly joking from bullying.

Barboa and Luck (2016) further maintained that communication is a key component of social interaction and is our most basic connection to other people. When the ability to communicate effectively (either through verbal or non-verbal means) is absent, it interferes with a functional and purposeful life. For children and adolescents with ASD, communication can be affected in many ways including:

- Lack of a social "filter"—the child or adolescent may say what they think even without understanding that the comment is inappropriate or offensive.

- Delays in language development.
- May be completely nonverbal.
- May lack ability to understand or express through body language.
- Exhibit repetitive speech, repeating phrases or complete scripts they have heard somewhere.
- May speak in a flat tone of voice.
- Difficulty constructing full sentences.
- May use sign language or an electronic communication device.
- May struggle with word choice and word meaning.
- Difficulty accurately expressing needs and wants.
- Struggles with receptive language—fully taking in and understating what is being said to them.

Dawson, McPartland, & Ozonoff (2002) stated that everyone diagnosed with ASD has trouble with social interchange, specifically with reciprocity, the back and forth interactions that make up all social encounters. Further, children and adolescents with ASD tend to have a very limited concept of friendship, tend to face peer rejection, and may struggle in initiating socially encouraging body language. When children and adolescents with ASD are placed in social situations where they do not have the proper social skills to maneuver the situation, it can create a great deal of anxiety for the child, which typically leads to unwanted behaviors. Just the thought of being put in a situation that is unfamiliar, or where there is a lack of skills to navigate successfully, can create a great deal of anxiety and lead to unwanted behaviors.

Dienstmann (2008) asserted that social skills must be taught. The belief that social skills magically appear in children without any development is a common misconception. Research supports social skills training as an evidence-based treatment for learning social skills. We know that social skills refer to many skills; from simple to complex. It is important to categorize social skills to better help identify individual skills that can be practiced during social group times. Some social skills are more foundational with other more complex skills building upon them. When working with children and adolescents to improve social skill deficits, it is critical to begin with skill deficits that are more basic or fundamental and advance to more complex skills. Table 2.1 provides a selection and categorization of some of the more common social skills with a formulated breakdown by level and complexity. The categorization guide does not necessarily flow sequentially. Many children will present with skill strengths and deficits throughout the guide. Levels four and five specially focus on emotional regulation and managing aggressive behavior. These are skills that would certainly be addressed continually and not something that would be paused until early level skills were acquired. The guide is a placement of social skills to help the therapist be more aware of the various social skills a child may need to improve. It demonstrates

Table 2.1 Social Skills Categorization Guide

Level 1	Level 2	Level 3	Level 4 (Level 4 specifically focuses on knowing and managing emotions)	Level 5 (Level 5 specifically focuses on alternatives for aggressive behavior)
Noticing Another Person	Asking For Help	Giving Instructions	Knowing Emotions	Avoiding Fights
Looking Toward People	Following Instructions	Convincing Others	Expressing Emotions Appropriately	Handling Anger-Related Feelings
Listening	Apologizing	Negotiating and Advocating	Recognizing Emotions in Others	Dealing with Accusation
Asking Questions	Asking Permission	Using Self Control	Expressing Concern for Others	Standing Up for Others
Starting a Simple Conversation	Sharing	Handling Bullying	Expressing Affection	Accepting No
Ending a Simple Conversation	Joining in a Group	Giving Compliments	Handling Anxiety	Relaxation Techniques
Saying Thank You	Helping Others	Accepting Consequences	Showing Compassion	Coping Skills
Introducing Self	Appropriate Body Language	Managing Disagreements	Emotion/Situation Appropriateness	
Introducing Other People	Appropriate Tone of Voice	Understanding Humor	Self-Regulation Ability	
Basic Acknowledgment of a Person	Understanding Personal Space	Recognizing Trouble Situations		
Basic Boundaries	Two-Way Conversation	Initiating Tasks		
Taking Turns	Making and Maintaining Friends	Completing Tasks Without Assistance		
	Public Boundaries	Well-Rounded Play Skills		
	Handling Winning and Losing	Problem Solving		
		Flexibility		
		Advanced Boundaries		

that some skills are more basic than others and, in some cases, there is a need to develop a lower-level skill before mastering a higher-level skill.

Before children or adolescents begin participating in a social skills group, it is essential to assess their current social skill strengths and deficits (Radley et al., 2016; Grant, 2017). For the group experience to be as smooth and successful as possible, it is essential that the children and adolescents participating be similar in their social skill strengths and deficits. If there exists too great a gap in social skills between the group members it will become challenging to improve social skills and may create further issues with children and adolescents being comfortable in the group. This could then affect group members' willingness to participate.

Any child or adolescent with ASD or related condition can participate in AutPlay social skills groups. The caveat is that children and adolescents around the same functioning and skill levels are placed in groups together. For example, four children ranging in age from four to six are participating in a play group together and they are all considered "high functioning" with verbal ability and interaction ability. We would not place a five-year-old in this group that was considered "low functioning," no verbal ability, no interaction skills. The "lower functioning" five-year-old would be in a group with two to three other children who were also considered "lower functioning" and assessed to be at about the same social skill level.

The process of assessing children and adolescents should take place prior to beginning a group. Parents should try to be forthcoming and aware of their child's strengths and deficits and share this information when discussing group participation. The AutPlay Social Skills Inventory (child and adolescent versions) provided in the Appendix of this book can be completed by parents to further identify their child's social skill strengths and deficits. Also provided in the Appendix section is the Group Readiness Questionnaire which explores more information about a child or adolescent and should also be completed prior to beginning a group. Both inventories will help identify children who are around the same functioning and social skill level. These inventories will guide the professional in placing children and adolescents in the most appropriate groups and also provide guidance on what skills to focus on for improvement and some general direction for group set up and process.

3 AutPlay® Therapy and Social Skills

Schaefer (2003) presented several therapeutic factors of play. He proposed that play helps in relationship enhancement, expressive communication, growth of competence, creative problem solving, abreaction, role play, learning through metaphor, positive emotion, and socialization. Children can learn social skills, develop relationships, learn how to communicate and express themselves through verbal and nonverbal means, and develop problem-solving abilities through therapeutic play.

The benefits of children engaging in play include cognitive development (learning, thinking, and planning, etc.), social skills (practicing social interaction, roles, and routines), language (talking to others, turn taking, etc.), problem solving (negotiation, asking for help, solving difficulties, etc.), and emotional development (managing feelings, understanding others, empathy, etc.). Children with adequate play skills are more likely to be included with their peers, and play is a key learning tool through which children develop social skills, flexibility, core learning skills, and language. Play also provides opportunities for children to practice events, situations, and routines in a safe place, with no pressure to "get it right" (Phillips and Beavan, 2010).

Although play has been established as a positive learning tool for children with ASD, there are play-related issues that are typical in children with autism. In general, children with ASD lack spontaneous, flexible, imaginative, and social qualities that are common with play. Playing with toys spontaneously, engaging in pretend and imaginative play, understanding metaphor in play, and successfully engaging in group play are typically skill deficits. Children with ASD are more likely to manipulate objects in a detached fashion rather than play symbolically. Cross (2010) listed five common play challenges that limit a child or adolescent with ASD's play potential and developmental skill acquisition:

1. Repetitious play.
2. Continual roaming around the playroom.
3. Continual anxiousness about or during play.
4. Continual detachment or unfriendliness during play.
5. Continual rejection by playmates during play.

When a child with ASD enters a playroom or any play environment, it is likely that he or she will not playfully engage in traditionally or socially deemed "correct" ways to play. A child with ASD might be very hesitant at first, taking a long time to get comfortable or familiar with what is around them, and then eventually engaging in some way; other children may isolate themselves and play with toys in a functional way, paying no attention to other people or things around them; some children may find an object not traditionally considered a toy but manipulate and "play" with the object while ignoring popular toys around them.

Children with ASD tend to have problems participating in social play with peers. Typically, children with ASD will become isolated in their play and withdraw from peer play groups. There is evidence to indicate that children with ASD do desire peer relationships and to participate in peer play but simply lack the social and communication skills to initiate and maintain such play. There is also evidence to indicate that children with ASD do indeed play and desire play. A child with ASD may play in non-traditional ways and may play with things that are not socially accepted as toys, but they do play (Grant 2017).

Each child with ASD or any developmental disorder will have a different placement in terms of play skills. The practitioner will often not know what level or ability of play the child is going to demonstrate. It is essential that proper assessment is done to see what play ability, level, or skill a child has. It is unfair to assume that every child with ASD will not have varied play skills. Some children with ASD will play, but in ways and with objects that may not seem like or look like traditional play. Some children with ASD do have advanced play skills and play skills that match their neurotypical peers. It is possible to have a child who is "higher functioning" on the autism spectrum who does engage in true pretend and imaginative play. It can be helpful to understand what typical compared to atypical play might look like in children. Table 3.1 provides Grant's (2017) guide for neurotypical verses atypical play in children.

There is little doubt that long-standing, developmentally based deficits in play and social function create significant lifelong disability. Deficits in social perception, social interest, social responsiveness, and atypical social communication and interaction patterns have a significant impact on children, adolescents, and adults with autism. Methods of play intervention that can reduce the impact of these deficits in a meaningful and sustainable way are of critical importance (LeGoff et al, 2014). AutPlay Therapy is an integrative family play therapy approach. It harnesses play to help children and adolescents affected by autism. AutPlay integrates behavioral therapy and play therapy theories such as Child Centered Play Therapy, Theraplay, Filial Therapy, and Cognitive Behavioral Play Therapy. AutPlay protocol includes evidence-based practices for working with autism. The approach includes play therapy interventions, parent training, and skill assessment.

Table 3.1 Neurotypical vs. Atypical Play in Children Ages Birth–10 yrs.

Neurotypical Play Development	Atypical Play Development
0–24 months A child explores the world through senses, mouthing objects, listening to sounds, looking at mobiles, etc.	Child does not explore, does not appear to notice, listen, or look at things. No shared cooing or smiling.
10 months Social reciprocal interaction begins, especially with parents, playing peek-a-boo with an adult.	Child does not interact, make eye contact, or engage in any basic interacting games.
1–2 years Imitates adults, then may imitate other children. May imitate mommy talking on the phone. Functional play emerges. Playing with a toy as it is intended to be played with, stacking blocks, rolling a car on a surface, etc.	Child does not speak, does not have joint attention, does not play with toys as they are supposed to be played with. Odd or no play. Does not play games with caregivers.
2–3 years Parallel play emerges. Playing side-by-side with a peer. Having the intention to be in proximity to peers during play. Child may play beside a familiar peer in a sand box. This starts with minimal verbal interaction with peers and gradually increases to watching and imitating peers, showing and commenting to peers, etc. Symbolic play emerges. Pretending with toys that look like real life objects, flying a toy airplane through the sky, pretending to cook with a pan on a play stove, pretending to eat play food, making people or animal figurines walk and talk.	Does not play with peers or show any interest in playing with peers, may not notice other peers. Does not do any imitation-based play. Does not do any pretend play. Continues to lack in playing with toys appropriately or engaging caregiver in basic play games.
3 years Play becomes more advanced and may involve peers and others more, may build and construct play objects (train sets, building houses, constructing Legos, making things out of play dough such as flowers, houses, faces, etc.). Child will engage in parallel, functional, and symbolic play often with other children but still may have difficulty with sharing and cooperative play. Role play and enactment emerges. Pretending to be familiar roles (such as teacher, doctor, bus driver, etc.).	Continues to not play with peers or show any interest in playing with peers. If playing with toys, may play with same toys over and over or line toys up continually. Does not do any symbolic play or role playing. Needs routine and predictability.

4 years

Role play and symbolic play become more and more advanced and children begin to learn how to play cooperatively. Pretend roles now may involve peers and still tend to be related to roles they have witnessed, whether in person, on TV, or in a book. Theory of mind emerges, the ability to consider that others have different thoughts, feelings, and knowledge than I do. Things can be other than what they seem, coinciding with development of more abstract play such as pretending a pencil is an airplane flying through the sky. Negotiation skills emerge as there is more awareness of other's desires and differences in thinking.

Child continues to lack symbolic and pretend play. Child continues to lack interest in playing with peers. Child will not play with peers in a cooperative fashion. Child shows no theory of mind concept. Child may focus on specific toys/items and be somewhat obsessive and rigid about the toy/item. If playing, may play with the same toy or play same scenario repeatedly.

5–6 years

Child may engage in complex play schemes with multiple other children. Involves all types of play, cooperating and negotiating with peers to develop play schemes and carry them out.

Child's play development has not increased from early developmental levels. Child is narrow in play interests and activities. Child continues to show no interest in playing with peers.

7–10 years

Child continues to develop more imaginative play, things that don't actually exist.

Child displays obvious play issues regarding all previously mentioned atypical play characteristics.

Grant (2017) stated that AutPlay Therapy is a combination of behavioral and relational approaches for working with children and adolescents with ASD, developmental delays, and other neurodevelopmental disorders. AutPlay addresses the skill development needs of children and adolescents affected by autism regardless of their impairment level. Protocol is designed to meet the child where he or she is in terms of ability and then address the child's specific needs. As a comprehensive model, the focus of AutPlay Therapy is to utilize the therapeutic powers of play to assist children and adolescents in gaining needed skills and abilities and to teach parents how to assist in becoming co-change agents in helping their children.

The AutPlay Therapy protocol can potentially incorporate and address any of the 20 core agents of change of the therapeutic powers of play presented by Schaefer & Drewes (2014). Therapeutic factors refer to specific clinical strategies, and therapeutic powers of play refer to the specific change agents in which play initiates, facilitates, or strengthens their therapeutic effect. The change agents include self-expression, access to the unconscious, direct teaching, indirect teaching, catharsis, abreaction, positive emotions, counterconditioning fears, stress inoculation, stress management, therapeutic relationship, attachment, social competence, empathy, creative problem solving, resiliency, moral development, accelerated psychological development, self-regulation, and self-esteem.

Through specific consideration and selection of the core change agents, children with ASD can learn social skills, develop relationships, learn how to communicate and express themselves through verbal and nonverbal means, improve emotional regulation ability, and develop problem solving abilities. AutPlay utilizes structured play therapy interventions that are specifically chosen and/or created for the individual child. Each intervention embodies one or more of the 20 core agents of change depending on the child's assessed needs. Although any of the core change agents could be identified and addressed with a child with ASD, typically children with an ASD diagnosis benefit from a focus on direct teaching, positive emotions, stress management, stress inoculation, empathy, therapeutic relationship, positive peer relationship, counterconditioning fears, social competence, and self-regulation (Grant 2019).

AutPlay Therapy incorporates a combination of directive play interventions with behavioral and play therapy approaches to teach children development in three primary target areas: emotional regulation, social functioning, and connection. AutPlay protocol also addresses three secondary target areas: sensory processing, anxiety reduction, and behavioral change. When children can learn to self-regulate, possess social skills that relate to the environments they are asked to function in, and learn appropriate and meaningful relationship connection, they are less likely to have behavioral issues and more likely to function successfully in their day-to-day environment (Grant 2017).

AutPlay Therapy teaches children with ASD social skills and functioning that is lacking in their current skill set. Children are first assessed to see what social skills they currently possess and what skills are in a deficit. Assessment is done by having parents and other caregivers complete the AutPlay Social Skills Inventory and by the professional conducting observations. Once an individual's social skill deficits have been assessed, directive play therapy interventions are chosen to work on each social skill that needs to improve. Children are taught social skills through several directive play therapy interventions that are done in the professional's office or play therapy room. The play therapy social skills interventions are then taught to the parents to practice with their child at home (Grant 2017).

A parent training component is incorporated into AutPlay Therapy where parents are trained in using various play therapy interventions at home with their child. Parents work with the AutPlay professional to help their child develop and advance in skill level. AutPlay Therapy's parent training component teaches parents how to conduct AutPlay interventions at home. Parents learn procedures and interventions and are shown how to implement interventions at home to increase specific skill and ability levels in their child. In AutPlay Therapy groups, parents become change agents for their children and play an integral role in the group process. Parents help their children and adolescents learn play and social skills and work directly with the professional.

Parent implemented intervention is an evidence-based practice for autism. Family members are typically present for a majority of the child's experiences and are the people in the child's life that remain constant while professionals are often transient. This level of social and familial consistency provides opportunity for parents to become effective change agents for their child. MacDonald and Stoika (2007) stated that the best place for children with ASD to learn language, relationship skills, social skills, and knowledge for everyday life is during their everyday life. There is no more meaningful time to teach language development, relationship skills, and social skills than while doing daily life together, and parents are typically the ones experiencing daily life with their child. AutPlay Therapy and AutPlay Therapy groups both include a parent training and implementation component. The specifics of parent involvement and training in AutPlay Therapy groups are further outlined in the following chapters.

AutPlay Therapy protocol is designed for any child or adolescent on the autism spectrum regardless of their severity level or functioning ability. Those who have a more severe impairment level or "lower functioning" ability participate in the AutPlay Therapy Follow Me Approach (FMA). This approach focuses on relationship development, skill development, and a movement for the child from an inability to focus and complete directive instruction to participating fully in professional and parent led directive play interventions. In FMA, the professional and child participate in a typical play therapy room. The child is given no directive instructions from the professional. The professional follows the child's lead, moving with the child around the room and trying to engage with the child in whatever activity they are doing. The professional lets the child lead but periodically tries to get involved with what the child is doing. The professional transitions as the child transitions. The professional is continuously looking for opportunities to connect with the child through eye contact, verbalizations, or any other engagement goals.

Throughout an FMA session, the professional is using reflecting and tracking statements while being mindful of the child's comfort level. In FMA, it is important to not only share physical space with the child, but also share attention, emotion, and understanding with the child. Initially, a child with ASD may find the FMA uncomfortable and the experience of someone trying to connect or engage with them intrusive. If a child starts to become agitated or dysregulated by the professional's attempts to get involved with what they are doing, then the professional should discontinue attempts to get involved and simply stay present with the child, providing reflecting and tracking statements. The professional may begin to reengage with the child once the child seems to feel comfortable. A typical session time with a child using FMA would last approximately 30 minutes. The remainder of the session should be spent processing with the parents. Parents are taught the AutPlay FMA. They observe several FMA sessions the professional conducts with the child and then transition to having FMA playtimes at home with their child.

There are two types of AutPlay groups—AutPlay Therapy play groups and AutPlay Therapy social skills groups. Both types of groups are further defined in the following chapters. AutPlay Therapy play and social skill groups follow the AutPlay Therapy protocol and design. There is a direct focus on utilizing the therapeutic powers of play with a special emphasis on improving social skill development. In AutPlay groups each child is assessed for skill strengths and deficits using AutPlay Therapy inventories. Parent involvement is emphasized in AutPlay groups as parents become co change agents in helping their child. Parents are taught play and social skill interventions and trained in facilitating social group meetings outside of the clinic. The basic dynamics of AutPlay Therapy serve to guide the formation and implementation of play and social skill groups.

4 AutPlay® Therapy Play Groups and Social Skills Groups

Implementing AutPlay Therapy groups requires therapists to be aware that some children will have a difficult time entering groups and engaging in play-based games and activities with their peers. This would be a logical reason that a child or adolescent would participate in a group—to become more proficient in peer interaction, play, and social skills. Emphasis should be placed on understating that these skills need practice and time to develop. For some children it may be necessary to begin working on social skills by meeting one on one with the professional and working toward joining a group. Professionals should use discretion when deciding if a child is ready for the type of group being offered. AutPlay Therapy play and social skill groups can be implemented for children across the spectrum regardless of their functioning ability, but the formation and implementation of the group can look differently depending on the impairment level of the group members. Therapists should consider the AutPlay Group Formation Guide (Table 4.1) when working with this population and establishing groups.

AutPlay Therapy groups provide a sense of belonging for children. Many children with autism and related conditions are left out of groups and activities that involve neurotypical peers. In AutPlay Therapy groups, children can develop relationships, practice skills, and have positive recreational experiences. Children and adolescents can gain a feeling of acceptance and optimism about social situations, especially social situations with peers. They may also discover they are not alone and that other peers have the same difficulties they do. AutPlay Therapy play and social skill groups should always provide:

- A safe and supportive environment for children and adolescents to interact.
- A natural and playful opportunity to learn and practice social skills.
- An opportunity to build self-esteem and confidence in social situations.
- An opportunity to establish friendships.
- A supportive environment for parents.

Table 4.1 AutPlay Group Formation Guide

- Decide on the age range and functioning level of group participants. The chronological age and the functioning level should be similar for group members.
- Decide how many participants will be in the group. Typically, six members would be a maximum. A group minimum for a group would be two participants. Some of this will be dictated by the functioning level of the participants (the more severe impairment, the fewer group participants) and the number of adults available to help facilitate the group (the fewer adults available, the fewer group participants). A typical guide would be to have one adult for every two group participants.
- Establish an assessment process to screen for similarities in functioning level and social skill deficits. It is better to have a group with children of similar ability levels and who need to work on similar social skills. The AutPlay Groups model provides an intake process to establish ability level and a social skills inventory to assess social skill deficits.
- Establish a screening process to assess for group readiness. Some children may not be ready to participate in a group format and will need to begin with individual therapy. The AutPlay groups model provides a group readiness form.

It is important to remember when working with any child and implementing play or any intervention, the professional will find that he or she participates at various levels with a child. This is determined by the professional when working with a child. If a child is more impaired and having trouble with a skill concept, the professional will become more involved and may lead most of the play or intervention, taking on more of an instructional and psychoeducational role. If a child is less impaired or more developed in a certain component, the professional will do less directing/instructing and will let the child create and develop in the play, intervention, or group process on their own. The professional will, at times, be very instruction/participant oriented, but the professional should always be looking for skill advancement in a child and challenging him or her to attempt more on their own.

The professional is the most important component of AutPlay Therapy groups. They are more valuable than any of the toys or interventions that might be used in the groups. Kottman (2011) described the four components of an Adlerian play therapist which parallel the role of professionals who facilitate AutPlay groups: (1) The professional is both a partner and encourager. (2) The professional is an active, relatively directive detective. (3) The professional is a partner, but also an educator. (4) The professional is an active teacher and encourager. These are certainly roles the professional facilitating an AutPlay group will find him or herself experiencing. Children and adolescents participating in AutPlay groups need facilitators who are flexible and adaptable; switching smoothly from child-led relationship building to psychoeducational teaching.

AutPlay Therapy interventions are often used in play and social skill groups. They are specifically designed to meet a child where he or she is at in terms of his or her level of play and social skill functioning. Aut-Play Therapy interventions help increase play and social functioning and other needed skills and abilities such as emotional regulation. AutPlay Therapy takes into account the lack of play and social skills that may be present in a child with ASD and introduces play and interventions in a specific manner so that children with ASD can participate and learn from them. Children and adolescents are thoroughly assessed at the beginning of group work to identify their skill deficits and assist the professional in creating treatment goals then choosing play interventions to specifically address each child's skill needs. The professional should implement play therapy interventions in groups using a simple three step guide:

1. Begin with simple play skill games and gradually build to more complex interventions. It is much easier to increase the level of an intervention than to correct for beginning above the participant's skill level.
2. Begin with play interventions that seem less threatening or anxiety producing and increase the variety of interventions as the group members' anxiety decreases.
3. Try to begin with interventions that are naturally engaging for the children in the group and build to more complex activities that require greater motivation on the part of the children.

When children and adolescents can develop better play and social skills, they can improve upon a whole host of skill deficits and keep improving throughout their lifetime. AutPlay Therapy groups utilize play and play related processes to help children and adolescents gain in social skill ability. For some children with ASD, play can look neurotypical, for others there may be play deficits such as an inability to implement pretend or symbolic play. AutPlay Therapy groups can help children and adolescents gain in play skills while simultaneously gaining in social ability. The utilization of play as a modality to teach social skills provides a natural and inviting atmosphere for all group members to participate.

Before starting a play or social skills group, there are a few things to consider. Children and adolescents with autism and other developmental disorders often thrive on structure, consistency, and predictability. In order to help increase more positive outcomes during group meetings, it will be very helpful for professionals to establish, from the beginning, how often they will meet, when and where they will meet, and how each meeting will be structured (suggestions are provided in the next chapter). To reduce dysregulation and ensure success, it will be especially helpful if professionals stay consistent and do not detour from the routine they have established with the group.

Relationship development is a critical feature when working with children with ASD and related conditions. The therapeutic relationship is a core change agent of play therapy and creates an atmosphere wherein children and adolescents can feel relaxed and confident to work on skill development. Therapeutic relationship development can be defined as purposeful positioning and response on the part of the professional that enables the child to feel safe, free to explore, express, and discover what the child needs in order to heal. It is a trusting process where the child believes the therapist is nonjudgmental, accepting, and can be trusted in the relationship. Children with autism are often anxious and even dysregulated by new people and environments. It is essential that therapists embody effective therapeutic relationship. Stewart & Echterling (2014) stated that when children are immersed in play activity, they lose their sense of self-awareness and they become caught up in the process. This experience of playful flow with the professional profoundly deepens and enriches the therapeutic relationship. The mindful process of the professional to stay present with the child, engaging in emphatic responding, provides an acceptance and nonjudgmental atmosphere, and communicates to the child that they are fully seen and heard. This defines the professional's movement in therapeutic relationship development in play. This process will greatly enable further exploration for all types of skill gain protocol.

Children and adolescents with developmental disorders need skill development work. Professionals will want to take note of the importance of addressing skill deficits with group goals including specific play and social skill gains. Structured play or interventions to address skill deficits can take on multiple forms. In general, some points to consider when using structured play or social skill interventions in AutPlay Therapy groups include the following:

1. Do not overthink it. It is not necessary to have an advanced social skills curriculum to implement solid, simple ideas to help teach social skills. Several interventions are provided in this book and professionals should remember to keep it focused on the play and social skill goals and not make things too complicated.
2. Do not try to do too much too soon. Again, keep it simple; focus on one skill and ways to learn that skill. Remember the shaping principal. Start with a small step and progressively move forward.
3. Children with developmental disorders are likely in environments where the focus is on structured teaching with little play or enjoyment. Avoid this atmosphere in AutPlay Therapy groups. Children will likely be more resistant, and less participation will be achieved if the group's atmosphere is too formal or rigid.
4. Keep the skill-learning component as natural as possible and incorporate it into the activity or play time that is planned. Integrate play

and a playful atmosphere. This will keep the children and adolescents engaged and relaxed so they can participate and gain the targeted skills.

5. Try to keep skill learning fun. Look for ways to add a fun element to every directive skill learning intervention. Structured play therapy interventions should be fun. The professional should try to keep the group process light and engaging even when implementing limits or providing redirection.

6. Remember that some social skills will be developed naturally simply by having the group meet together even if no structured social skill interventions are presented.

7. Remember that developing social skills takes time. Some children in the group may develop skills more quickly than others. There is no limit to how long a social skills group can meet, and it would be expected to see children with developmental disorders gain skills at different rates.

8. Professionals are strongly encouraged to use the resources section at the end of this book which provides several publications and websites where parents can find more activities, techniques, and games that can be integrated into AutPlay Therapy play and social skill groups. Although this book includes several interventions for increasing social skills, professionals can access more interventions and activities to have a wide variety from which to choose.

Handling Unwanted Behavior

When a group of children or adolescents with autism or other developmental disorders come together, there is always potential for dysregulation and possible negative behaviors. Handling situations where a child is having a "meltdown" or having behavior that has become unsafe for themselves or others around them, should be done with care and support.

In AutPlay Therapy play and social skills groups, there is no judgment or penalty if at any time the child needs to leave the group. This may be to take a break and then return before the group session ends, it may mean skipping a session, or it may mean that the child discontinues with the group at this time. This should be at the child and professional's discretion and parents should provide support as needed. If a child is having behavior that is disruptive or unsafe, it could be helpful for professionals to establish in advance an exit or break routine that minimizes disruption for the rest of the group and helps facilitate a positive return to the group. An example of this could be a code word that alerts the regulated group members to stand up and walk to another room while the professional diffuses the disruption. If a child leaves the group meeting for that day, the child should return to the next scheduled meeting unless another decision has been made.

Professionals should not be disturbed by conflicts that may occur in groups. Some conflict is natural and occurs with all children. Professionals should look at conflicts as learning opportunities that can ultimately help children develop social skills. Some children may have several meltdowns during several meetings. This is a part of the process; the child is learning how to be in social environments. Some possible scenarios include adjusting a child's participation time, such as participating thirty minutes for several meetings instead of one hour and working their way up to more time. Having a separate break room available that a child can go to if they are needing a break from the group, adjusting so the child participates in every other group session instead of every session, providing a particular child a one-on-one support person to assist them through group time, or discussing with the parent and child that the child may not be ready for a group and agreeing to see the child individually for therapy and working toward participating in a group.

No child or parent should be penalized for a child's behavior. AutPlay Therapy play and social skill groups are not only skill groups, but support groups that are inclusive and never should they be rejecting. I am reminded of a good friend's story about her daughter participating in a social skills group marketed and designed for children with ASD. An autism clinic was facilitating the group with trained autism specialists. My friend wanted her daughter to participate in the group in hopes that her daughter's social skills would improve. A few group sessions into the process, the facilitators asked this mother to not bring her daughter back because her daughter was too disruptive and did not possess the social skills to participate in the group at that time. If a social skills group is not for children who really need help with social skills, then who are these groups for? This story illustrates the opposite of what AutPlay Therapy play and social skills groups promote. No child should ever simply be removed from an AutPlay Therapy group. No parent or child should ever experience this type of rejection. AutPlay Therapy groups are about accepting, learning, supporting, and growing together. Talking with a child and parent about leaving the group should be a last resort and should always accompany a new plan for the child such as working with them individually.

Most behavior that will occur in a group will likely be the result of the child being dysregulated. A hallmark issue in children with autism and related conditions is easily becoming dysregulated. Children with autism frequently lack the skill ability to modulate their emotions and regulate through situations that are causing them distress. A child could become dysregulated due to being exposed to a new environment, having their routine changed, lacking social skills to navigate situations, inability to appropriately express emotions, lack of coping skills, high anxiety, sensory processing struggles, etc. Many things can cause a child to become dysregulated and once the child is in a dysregulated state, they are unable to control their behavior.

There is a time frame before a child has crossed into a full-blown dysregulated state, that interventions may help to provide regulation and prevent the child from becoming more dysregulated. If the professional can identify when a child starts to become dysregulated, the professional can assist the child in regulation interventions and likely prevent a meltdown. Once a child has crossed over into a full-blown meltdown, there is very little that can be done to stop the process. Most children will need to be guided to a safe place and left alone with no sensory input. Once they have calmed, the professional can talk with them and create strategies to try and prevent the dysregulation from happening again. Often simply providing a break option and/or access to some regulation/sensory materials can help the child calm, regulate, reset, and return to the group. In certain groups, the professional may decide to complete a brief regulation activity with all of the group members, making the assumption that all of them may feel a bit dysregulated. This may reduce more severe meltdowns later on during the group session.

Limit Setting Models

Occasionally behavior that happens in a group will need to be addressed in the moment. There are several limit setting models in play therapy that would be appropriate to use. Regardless of the model chosen, the professional should be consistent with implementation. Typically play therapy limit setting models are not pre-explained to children, but in AutPlay Therapy groups it is important to explain to the group in the first session what the expectations are for behavior and treating/interacting with others. The professional should also explain the limit setting model that will be used and provide examples.

The AutPlay Therapy limit setting model (Grant, 2017) provides one option for managing unwanted or disruptive behavior. The three R's limit setting model stands for redirect, replacement, and removal. The professional may implement a redirect or a replacement at any time, choosing one or the other or trying both. Removal is a final step and should only be used as a last resort.

> *Redirect*—If the child begins to or is breaking a limit, the professional should start with redirection. The professional or parent would simply try to redirect the child to another activity, toy, or object to transition their attention off the limit violation. There does not need to be any dialogue about a limit being broken or that the child needs to stop, but it is recommended to add a simple verbal prompt such as "In here we cannot do that." The professional realizes the limit is being broken and moves to see if redirecting will suffice.
>
> *Replacement*—If the child begins or is in process of breaking a limit, the practitioner or parent can begin with redirecting the child or

begin with replacement. These two processes can be used inter-changeably. Replacement means literally replacing what is happening with something new or different. If for example, the child is smashing a toy truck into the floor which is breaking the truck, the professional would quickly select another object such as a rubber ball and put it in the child's free hand while taking the truck away from the child. Replacement can also be replacing a game that is being played by the child with a different game. Where redirection is the act of transitioning the child's attention or trying to distract the child away, replacement is giving the child a tangible, acceptable alternative. As with redirecting, there does not need to be any dialogue about the limit being broken when using the replacement strategy, but it is recommended to add a simple verbal prompt letting the child know the behavior cannot be done in the playroom.

Removal—If a child is beginning to or in the process of breaking a limit, redirecting and replacement should be implemented first. If these processes do not work, then removal is the final option. The first step in removal is verbally explaining to the child that they need to discontinue a behavior, or they may be removed from the room. If the verbal prompt does not stop the behavior, then removal is implemented. Removal is guiding the child into another location, possibly where the child can be alone or minimally supervised while the child calms. In an extreme case, removal might involve physically taking the child to a more secure location. If physical removal is necessary, then parents should be the person to physically remove the child. This is done in extreme cases where the child or others are in danger due to the child's behavior, and action is needed to keep everyone safe. Removal may also include moving the other group members to a safe location if the child in question is having severe dysregulation.

Landreth (1991) proposed the ACT limit setting model in Child Centered Play Therapy and stated that limits provide structure for the development of the therapeutic relationship and help to make the experience a real-life relationship. Without limits a relationship would have little value. The ACT limit setting model contains three steps and can be used when a therapist feels that a limit needs to be addressed in a group. The professional can repeat the three-step model for any limit and use this model as a primary for addressing limits if the group participants seem to adhere to the model.

Step One: A—Acknowledge what the child wants or needs or is feeling.
Step Two: C—Communicate the limit in a non-punitive manner.
Step Three: T—Target acceptable alternatives which the child could do.

An example of using the ACT limit setting model in an AutPlay group would be if one of the participants is throwing Legos at other participants and around the room. The professional would say (A) "Michael, I know you want to throw the Legos, (C) but in here we cannot throw Legos; (T) you can throw those soft balls to another person or you can build with the Legos." The limit can be stated very quickly, and the child should be given a moment to process what they have heard and correct their behavior. The limit can be repeated if the child continues with the behavior. If the child continues and does not adhere to the limit, on the third time, the therapist can say "if you choose to continue throwing the Legos, you are choosing to take a break from the group or even end your group time today." It is up to the therapist what the final "consequence" will be. Therapists should try giving the statement that a problem item (Legos) will be removed and then removing the item first, but ultimately the therapist may have to state that the group session will end for that individual if they choose to continue to break the limit. If the therapist has made one of these statements and the child continues breaking the limit, the therapist must follow through and send the child to a break time or end their time in the group for that session.

VanFleet (2014) stated that limit setting in Filial Therapy provides children with boundaries that are essential to their sense of security. Limit setting helps children learn that they are responsible for what happens if they choose to break a limit. The Filial Therapy limit setting model contains a three-step sequence. The professional states the limit, gives a warning, and enforces the consequence. The professional would make a statement such as "one of the things you cannot do in here is paint on the wall, but you can do just about anything else." This is a simple statement that can be made very quickly. It can be repeated for any limits that need to be addressed. If the child continues to break the same limit, the professional repeats the statement and now adds a warning such as "Remember I told you that you could not paint on the walls. If you paint on the walls again, I will end your group time today." If the child continues to break the limit, the professional initiates the third step in the three-step sequence which is implementing the consequence. The professional would remind the child of the limit and the warning and state, "We must now end your group time for today."

The Filial Therapy limit setting model can be very effective for children and teens with ASD as it is simple and not too cognitive. The limit can be stated clearly and there is a direct behavioral consequence if the limit continues to be broken. This limit setting model could be used as the primary approach for addressing unwanted behaviors in the group setting if the participants responded well to the model. If a child reaches the point of ending their time in the group, one of the adults should escort the child out of the group and to their parent. There is no need for further dialogue or for the child to have a consequence at home. The child can return to the next group meeting.

In Adlerian Play Therapy, limit setting is designed to enhance the child's self-control and teach them that they have the ability to consider alternative behaviors and to redirect their own inappropriate behaviors (Kottman, 2003). When implementing the limit setting model, therapists must remain calm and communicate to the child confidence that the child will be able to follow the limit and change their behavior. The limit setting model comprises four steps—stating the limit, reflecting the child's feelings, generating acceptable alternatives, and logical consequences. For example, the therapist might say, "The rule in the group is that you cannot touch another person." "I can tell you are frustrated, but we need to keep our hands to ourselves." "Other group members are not for hitting, but I bet you can think of some things you can hit in the group room that would be OK."

There are several possible ways the Adlerian limit setting model could be stated. Many different phrases could be used depending on the child and the limit issue. The goal is to work with the child in having the child understand the limit and resolve the issue with an acceptable solution. If the child continues to break the limit, the fourth step is initiated which is giving a logical consequence. This is designed to encourage responsible behavior. This is ideally formulated with the child's input to establish a respectful and meaningful consequence for the limit that was broken. This limit setting model is very thorough and is somewhat of a process. It may be too verbal or too cognitive for more severely impaired children but could be very useful for children with ASD who have a higher functioning ability and better executive functioning skills.

Parent and Family Involvement

Social skills interventions have been found to result in limited generalization of skills across people and settings. Whereas individuals with ASD may demonstrate improvements in skill use within a training environment, effects are often more limited in naturalistic settings. The lack of generalized effects of social skills training may, in part, be a result of factors such as training in contrived settings (e.g., pull-out social skills groups) or lack of programming for generalization. Thus, to promote generalization of social skills, it is important that social skills training incorporate natural stimuli into the training environment (e.g., setting, peers), allow for participants to demonstrate social skill learning in more natural scenarios, and train diversely and loosely (Murphy et al., 2017).

Incorporating parents into AutPlay groups helps address issues of generalization and provides for more naturalist opportunity to implement and practice play and social skills. Parents participate in AutPlay play groups by spending time in the group playing with their child and other children.

Parents are then taught to create opportunities between group sessions to help their child implement the play and social skills they are learning in the group setting. This is in the form of setting up play dates with other children or going to a park or public play area and allowing their child to interact with other children and practice the play skills they have been learning in the group. Parents participate in AutPlay social skills groups by hosting a "hang out" time for all the group members every other week. This gives the group participants an opportunity in a more naturalist setting to practice the skills they have been learning in the group.

More details are provided in the following chapters on the pragmatics of how parent training and involvement is established in AutPlay groups. The nature of involvement will expose parents to other parents and to other children with autism. Participating in AutPlay groups provides the opportunity for parents to work directly with the professional and their child to help their child gain play and social skills. Participation also provides the opportunity for parents to spend meaningful time with their child. It's not unusual for parents to report they feel like they are having play times for the first time with their child.

The design of AutPlay groups creates several scenarios where parents will be exposed to and interacting with other parents and children. Parents should focus on being supportive with other parents and children, avoiding judgmental comments or actions, and focusing on helping and learning from interacting with one another. The professional will want to stress a collaborative and nonjudgmental process to parents, as there could be issues that parents disagree about or behaviors that each parent would handle differently. Any substantial issue or disagreement should be brought to the professional to mediate. As parents participate in the group process, it can expose different issues which the professional will want to address.

Working with children with developmental disorders is going to involve behavior issues. Each child in the group will likely, at times, display unwanted or problematic behavior. Parents should not be embarrassed by their child's behavior and not allow the behavior to cause them stress. The professional should discuss with the parents strategies and ideas presented in this book for handling unwanted behavior and implementing limit setting models. If needed, parents can also meet one on one with the professional to discuss behavior management ideas. It's important for parents to support other parents when their child is having behavior issues and not be judgmental or accusing. Each child is participating in the group because each child needs to work on more appropriate social interaction. It's necessary to convey to parents that this is collaborative process designed to help each child in the group improve social skill difficulties.

AutPlay groups ask parents to participate on a weekly basis and implement protocols at home outside of the group meeting. Parents should not feel overloaded or overwhelmed with group participation. The professional should discuss with parents how to manage their schedule and what level of participation with the group they feel they can manage. Parents are encouraged to take breaks as needed and work with their child at their own pace. AutPlay groups function better with parent involvement. It's critical that parents participate at a level that feels comfortable to them. If parents feel too burdened by group participation, it is likely they will leave the group. If needed, the therapist can meet one on one with a parent to discuss their level of participation and self-care strategies. Parents should be reminded that they are the most important relationship in their child's life. Participation in play and social skill groups increases healthy relationship development between the parent and child. Relationship development also provides the catalyst for children to cooperate more fully with their parents, engage more actively in directive social skill experiences, and provide confidence for the child to explore social skill growth.

AutPlay play and social skill groups focus primarily on helping children and adolescents learn play and social skills, but an indirect benefit of such groups is the parent support that is created. Parents with children who have autism, or related disorders understand and know better than anyone else what other parents with a child with ASD are questioning, struggling with, and worrying about. AutPlay groups provide parents the chance to be with other parents, share with them, learn from them, and gain support. The parent support aspect of AutPlay groups should not be undervalued. Often, parents are searching for a parent support group to share with, learn from, be accepted by, and generally feel a sense of community and understanding. The support and benefits that can materialize from a group of parents coming together and working collaboratively to increase skill development in their children is invaluable.

Parents play a critical role in helping their child successfully implement new play and social skills across environments. At times, parents themselves may lack critical social skills and may not have a full understanding of why their child needs to participate in a group or how the process is going to help their child. The professional may need to provide psychoeducation to the parents about how AutPlay groups can help improve play and social skills and how this directly affects improvement in unwanted behavior (Mellenthin, 2018). Professionals must be prepared to conceptualize not just the child participant but also the parent as a client and consider both part of the therapeutic group process.

Ethical Considerations in AutPlay Therapy Groups

Ethical considerations for group processes are not necessarily based in any group therapy protocol but rather on the ethical guidelines established by licensing boards and governing mental health organizations. Professionals should take care to familiarize themselves with best practices and ethical guides highlighted by their specific state licensing boards. The Association of Play Therapy (APT) outlines in their Play Therapy Best Practices (2019) considerations for play therapists conducting group work:

> The play therapist selects clients for group play therapy whose needs are compatible and conducive to the therapeutic process and well-being of each client. Play therapists using group play therapy take reasonable precautions in protecting clients from physical and psychological trauma. Play therapists explain to group members, and/or their legal guardians (when the group includes those who are legally under guardianship) the importance of maintaining confidentiality outside of the group, instruct them in methods for doing so and make special efforts to ensure confidentiality in settings where it may be more readily compromised, such as schools or inpatient/residential treatment settings. Rules for the group and consequence of breaking the rules should be clear to all group members. If a member of the group cannot abide by the rules of the group, consequences need to be enforced for the protection of others.
>
> (p. 6)

Further, the APT Best Practices guide highlights information regarding informed consent and confidentiality:

> Play therapists inform clients and/or their legal guardian when applicable, of the purposes, goals, techniques, procedural limitations, potential and foreseeable risks, risks of inconsistent compliance, and benefits of the services to be performed. This information will be provided in developmentally (and culturally) appropriate language for the understanding of the client and their legal guardian. Play therapists take steps to ensure that clients, and their legal guardian when applicable, understand the implications of diagnosis, treatment modalities, treatment interventions, the intention of assessment and reports, and fees and billing arrangements. Clients have the right to expect confidentiality and to be provided with an explanation of its limitations, including disclosure to appropriate legal guardian(s), disclosure as legally required and for safety when an immediate safety risk is revealed, suspicion of child abuse or other safety issue, supervision and/or treatment team case reviews, and requests made by the payer, and/or governmental authority and/or by court order to obtain information about any documents or documentations in their case records. Play therapists seek legal guardian's signature on all consents, including for treatment whenever applicable and when not constricted by state and/or federal laws and their legal and ethical codes of their license and professional organization.
>
> (p. 4)

In AutPlay Therapy groups, one of the primary areas to address is confidentiality. Because of the nature of parent involvement in the group process, children and parents will be exposed to other children and parents and will likely be aware of information about the other children and parents. Professionals cannot guarantee that group participants will maintain confidentiality and privacy of other group participants. The importance of maintaining confidentiality should be communicated to the group (Sweeney et al, 2014). The AutPlay professional must stress to group participants (children and parents) the importance of maintaining confidentiality and that, due to the nature of being involved in a group, confidentiality cannot be guaranteed. There should be a process established by the professional (which should be shared with group participants) outlining the consequences when group confidentiality and privacy are broken. The process of maintaining confidentiality and adherence to keeping information private should be outlined in the informed consent document that parents must sign prior to beginning the group process.

5 AutPlay® Therapy Play Groups (10-Session Model)

Play therapy groups developed in part because patterns of behavior emerged in children in group environments that were not present in the play of individual children. Groups focusing on children have grown in the past decade. Professionals have discovered that processes in groups cannot be replicated in individual work, and the group atmosphere holds much benefit for children (Knell, 1997). Groups serve as a practice field for the outside world, and the expressive and projective nature of play groups enable this practice to become real, thus easier to transfer and generalize to other settings and experiences (Sweeney et al, 2014).

AutPlay play groups are based off of the Follow Me Approach (FMA) in AutPlay Therapy. The FMA is used with children who have a functioning level that creates issues with focusing on and being able to participate in directive play therapy interventions, as well as children who are too young to participate in directive interventions. While this may often be younger children, play groups can apply to older children or adolescents. The FMA focuses on relationship development, skill development, and a movement for the child from an inability to focus and complete directive instruction to participating fully in professional and parent led directive play interventions (Grant 2017).

In FMA, the professional and child participate in a typical play therapy room environment. The child is given no directive instructions from the professional other than a structuring statement to begin the session such as, "This is the playroom, and you can play with anything you want and I will be in here with you." The professional follows the child's lead, moving with the child around the playroom and trying to engage with the child in whatever activity or toy he or she is playing with. The professional lets the child lead but always tries to get involved with what the child is doing. The professional transitions as the child transitions and is continuously looking for opportunities to connect with the child through eye contact, verbalizations, or any other play and social goals that are being targeted. As the child transitions from one toy or activity to another, the professional transitions with the child.

Table 5.1 AutPlay Follow Me Approach (FMA) Components

1. Follow the Child—The child leads, and the professional follows the child figuratively and literally. The professional lets the child move around the playroom and lets the child play with anything that he or she wants. The professional moves with the child, sits by the child, and transitions as the child transitions.
2. Make Tracking Statements—These are statements that the professional makes periodically tracking what the child is doing. For example: "You are playing in the sand tray," or "You just shot the Nerf gun," or "You are looking around at all the toys in here."
3. Make Reflecting Statements—These are statements that the professional makes when the professional notices the child displaying a feeling. For example: "That makes you mad," or "You feel sad that there is no more paint."
4. Ask Questions—The professional should periodically ask the child questions. The professional should try to ask questions that are relevant. For example: The child picks up a basketball. The professional might ask, "Do you have a basketball at home?"
5. Attempt to Engage with the Child—The professional should frequently try to engage the child or play with the child in whatever he or she is doing. For example: The child is playing in the sand tray. The professional might try scooping up some sand and pouring it on the child's hand or scooping up some sand and putting it in the bucket the child is trying to fill. Another example: The child is playing with some balls; the practitioner might pick up a ball and try to roll it or toss it to the child.
6. Introduce Simple Directive Games—The professional should periodically introduce a simple directive game or activity to see if the child will participate with the professional. This is somewhat of a "testing out" process to evaluate if the child is making progress toward participating in more reciprocal social play.
7. Be Mindful of Goals—The professional is constantly monitoring the child's play, social interaction, and engagement ability with others and taking note of progress and advancements in skill development.

Throughout the FMA session, the professional is using reflecting and tracking statements and being mindful of the child's comfort level. In the FMA, it is important to not only share physical space with the child, but also share attention, emotion, and understanding with the child. Parents are taught how to have FMA play times at home with their child and thus become co-change agents in helping their child develop skills. Table 5.1 highlights the key principles in the FMA which are the basic roles of the professional when implementing AutPlay play groups.

AutPlay play groups are typically designed for preschool-aged children because of their age and the more natural medium of play to be used in helping these children gain in social play skills. AutPlay play groups could be used with older children and adolescents who are more severely impaired or have a lower-functioning ability, as play would likely be the most successful medium for participation and growth. AutPlay play groups may also be useful for older children who may have a higher functioning ability but are highly resistant to participating in directive play interventions. In these situations, a less-directive play group may be more appropriate.

Pragmatics of AutPlay Play Groups

Definition of AutPlay Play Groups—These groups are designed for preschool aged children who have a diagnosis of autism or related condition. They are also appropriate for children of other ages who are struggling with social interaction. AutPlay play groups provide an atmosphere of playful interaction facilitated by a professional and includes parent participation.

Role of the Professional—The professional organizes and facilitates the play group process. The professional is a player and an encourager for both the children and the parents. Often, the professional serves as a role model and a teacher. The professional is active in the play groups by attempting to engage and play with children, establishing limits when necessary, and providing examples of social play strategies to parents.

Structure—AutPlay play groups are typically 50 minutes and consist of 20 group sessions. The group begins with a meeting in the professional's clinic where children participate in a play group (this typically occurs in a playroom or designated play space). The next week, the group participants meet together outside of the clinic to have a less formal play date meeting. This meeting is hosted by one of the participant's parents. The meetings alternate in this fashion weekly for 20 meetings—10 in clinic play meetings and 10 outside play date meetings. A step-by-step organization and structure guide for starting an AutPlay play group is provided in the appendix section of this book.

Generating Interest in a Group—Professionals should assess their local community for the need for play groups. This can be done by contacting local agencies that work with young children with ASD, contacting early intervention programs, contacting special needs preschools, and checking with local parent support groups.

Organization of a Group—The professional should decide on a possible start date and location for the group. The professional should also prepare any forms needed for the group and begin to market the group. A sample marketing flier is provided in the appendix section of this book.

Assessing/Screening Group Members—It is important that group members are as similar as possible when it comes to age and developmental level. Gender tends to not be as important as having children in the same group who are at about the same functioning level. When you have groups with many ages and several different functioning levels, you lose some of the environmental conditions that help develop social skills. The Intake Form and Group Readiness Questionnaire found in the appendix section of this book can be used to help assess group participants.

The professional should meet with each parent and child who might be interested in participating in a play group. This meeting is an opportunity to complete necessary documents, assess the child's ability level, and decide if the child would be an appropriate fit for the group that is beginning. If the child is assessed to not be ready for a group experience, the professional should try to offer meeting with the child for individual therapy and working toward joining a group. The professional can offer more than one group. This might be especially helpful if there are children of different developmental levels wanting to attend—the professional could offer multiple groups, matching the children with the best fit group. It might be necessary to place some children on a group wait list until there are enough children interested in participating in a group that are at the same developmental level. AutPlay play groups are focused on preschool-aged children so the age will not vary much in the participants, but professionals will want to pay close attention to the developmental and functioning levels of potential participants as these areas might vary considerably.

Who Can Participate—Any preschool aged child can participate in an AutPlay play group. Participants do not need a formal diagnosis of autism. Although a primary focus of the group is ASD issues, any child who might benefit from the play and social work of the group could participate.

Group Size—The typical size of a group should be four to five children, with no more than six. Anything larger will negatively affect the ability of the group to naturally connect and work on social play skills. Groups can be smaller and still be beneficial, but larger groups should be avoided. It would likely be better to have two groups of three than one group of six. The minimum number of participants for a group is two. Professionals should strive for a ratio of one adult for every two children, so the larger the group size, the more adults that will be needed to facilitate the group. These are recommendations for group size. This will vary depending on the functioning level of the participants. It might be possible for one professional to work with a group of three children if they were older children and their functioning ability was high. Likewise, if the participants are more severely impaired, the group may require a one-to-one ratio of child to adult.

Length of Group Meetings—The length of time a group meets may vary depending on the professional's preference, but the group structure for AutPlay play groups is based on a 50-minute group session. Some professionals may prefer to lengthen or shorten the group time.

Number of Group Meetings—AutPlay play groups meet for 10 in-clinic, more formal play times and 10 less formal play date times outside of the clinic. This is a total of 20 meetings. The formal and informal meetings alternate week to week. The first week the group meets in the clinic, the next week they meet outside of the clinic. The professional does not attend the outside-of-clinic meetings; these are hosted by one of the participant's parents. The professional can begin new groups at any time or start another group when one ends, and the new groups can include some of the same participants from a previous group. It is important to formally end a group after the 20 meetings to give children and parents a clean opportunity to leave the group.

Play Development—Since much of the group focus will be on play, it is important to assess each child's play skills and deficits. The AutPlay Groups Assessment of Play form is provided in the appendix section of this book. The professional will give the parent the assessment form to complete as part of the group intake process prior to the group beginning.

Social Skill Development—AutPlay play groups provide an integrative process of clinical and natural opportunity for children and adolescents to develop play and social skills. A more formal play time happens in the clinic meetings while a less formal, more naturalist process happens during outside of the clinic meetings. Both experiences are important for children with ASD to gain play and social skills. In AutPlay play groups, play is the process by which children begin to development more peer interaction social skills. The play process (outlined in Chapter 4) facilitates the acquisition of age appropriate social skills, especially those related to social interaction and peer play.

Group Meeting Locations—The professional will likely have in-clinic meetings at his or her clinic or some arranged meeting place. It is ideal for the in-clinic meeting location to be in a playroom or an established play space and to stay consistent throughout the duration of the group. For the parent-hosted, outside-the-clinic play dates, there are many options where a group could meet (this is typically decided on by the parent who is hosting). A common setting, such as a parent's home, a church, or a support group meeting facility, would certainly work. It is highly encouraged that some of the play date meetings occur in public. This may be a certain event, or specific activity designed for children; it may simply be going to a restaurant or park. Some parents may need help in deciding where to meet. Table 5.2 provides some meeting place options for parents. Also, the professional should communicate to

Table 5.2 Meeting Places for Parent-Hosted Play Groups

Parent's Home	Park
Kids Play Place	Public Library
Pet Store	Kids Play Place
Kids Museum	School Playground
Restaurant Play Area	Petting Zoo

parents that the parent-hosted play dates should not include any formal social skills interventions. This is a time for the participants to be together and practice natural social play. The parents can help their child to interact but there should be no pressure or purposeful teaching. The participants need this time to be with other children and enjoy a group social play experience.

It is helpful for parents to understand the dynamics of the children in the group and where each child is at in terms of functioning level and tolerance for certain situations. It is equally important for parents to know of particular issues with each child, such as any sensory issues, allergies, medical conditions, or fears related to certain environments. Any information about any of the group participants that would guide the selection of location or event for a parent hosted play date should be shared with the parents to avoid any potential issues. Where to meet and the type of play experience should be decided on and communicated the week before the parent hosted play date. Typically, the professional will have this information and share it with all the children and parents at the end of the in-clinic meeting. This information is included on the Session Overview Form (located in the appendix section) that is given to the parents at the end of each in-clinic meeting.

Handling Unwanted Behavior—The professional will want to choose one of the limit setting models defined in this book and explain the limit setting model to the parents and children during the first meeting. Modeling and practicing the limit setting model during this meeting may also be beneficial for the parents and children. The professional should use the limit setting model consistently. Each model provides for a final consequence of ending the group time for the child if the behavior does not change and/or is too disruptive. The professional should be patient and implement limits at a minimum. It is expected that there will be some unwanted and troublesome behavior. This should be relayed to all of the parents, so they are not surprised when it happens. If it is something the professional can work with and correct easily, then there is no need for further consequence. Some children may become dysregulated by being around other children. If possible, providing children the opportunity to move to a location in the playroom and play alone for a while can be helpful. Providing a break from the interaction can help children regulate and manage through the play group experience.

When parents are hosting a play date, the professional will not typically be present. The parents may need some brief instruction on how to handle unwanted behavior. This is more fully explained in Chapter 4. Professionals can teach the parents limit setting models and other interventions. It's important to explain to parents that behaviors will likely occur during a parent hosted meeting. If a parent has certain strategies they typically implement to help their child calm, the parent should implement these strategies. If a parent feels like they need to leave the play date this is Ok. The parent and child should leave, and they can try again at the next meeting. Other parents should get involved only if the parent of the child having unwanted behavior asks for assistance. It is important that the parent of the child having the unwanted behavior is the primary person addressing their child and trying to manage the behavior.

Parents as Co-Change Agents—Parents participate in AutPlay play groups. In the AutPlay Therapy Follow Me Approach (FMA), parents work with the professional in learning how to have special play times at home with their child. In AutPlay play groups, parents host a play date meeting outside of the clinic to help further the acquisition of social play gains. This process is fully explained to parents during the initial consultation about the play group. Any training, suggestions, or help a parent may need should be provided by the professional. If a parent has concerns and would like suggestions for hosting a group time, the professional should meet with the parent and provide the information they are requesting. The professional should communicate to parents that they are an important part of the play group process and empower parents to feel confident in their participation.

When parents host a play date meeting, the other parents should participate in each group meeting as much as possible. It may not be necessary for every parent to be at every meeting if parents are comfortable with others taking care of their children (this will depend on the size of the group and the developmental and functioning level of group participants). It is important that there are enough parents at each group meeting to care for the children and facilitate the group. Play groups provide a good opportunity for parents to socialize and find support, thus it is recommended that parents participate with their children as often as they can.

10-SESSION GUIDE FOR IN CLINIC AUTPLAY PLAY GROUPS

Play Group Session One

Note: Professionals should review the step-by-step guide for beginning an AutPlay group. This is located in the appendix section of this book.

Length

Based on a 50-minute group session.

About This Week's Group

The professional should take note of any specific information they want to cover or address in this group session. The professional should review and prep for the session time. Are there any specific toys or materials that need to be highlighted? Does the room need any adjustments? Is the Session Overview Form for parents completed and ready to give to parents? During the first session the children will follow the professional out of the waiting room and into the playroom. Parents will remain in the waiting room until they join the group with about 20 minutes left.

The Table

This is typically a literal table (usually a small child's table with chairs) but could also be a space on the floor, perhaps a blanket put down on the floor. This is for displaying selected toys or materials designed to promote social interaction. In AutPlay play groups the children are free to roam the playroom or play space and play with anything they want but sometimes, the professional may want to place specific toys or materials on the "Table" to promote children playing together. Utilizing the "Table" concept is optional and may not be done in each session but should be considered as another tool to help promote social play.

Structuring Statement

Once the professional has greeted everyone in the waiting room and all the children are in the playroom, the professional will make a simple structuring statement—"This is the playroom and you can play with anything you want in here and I (we) will be in here with you." Nothing else needs to be said or explained to the children at this time.

Play and Social Time

The children will have 35 minutes of unstructured play time. They may play with anything they want, and the professional(s) will move around the playroom making tracking and reflective statements and trying to encourage interactive play with themselves and other children in the group. The professional is not aggressive and does not force any child to interact or play with anyone else. The professional makes consistent attempts and encourages but allows the process to develop at the child's comfort level.

Parent and Child Play Time

Parents join the group for the last 20 minutes. One of the professionals will get the parents from the waiting room when there is about 20 minutes left of the group time. Once the parents are in the playroom, they are given the following directive: "This is your time to play and interact with your child or any other parent and child, and we will be in here with you." This is an opportunity for the professional to further observe the parent/child interaction, role model play attempts with the child, and allow for more social play experiences.

Five Minute Warning

When there is around five minutes left of the group time, the professional will make the following statement "We have five minutes left of our group time today, then it will be time to go." The professional makes another statement when there is one minute left of group time—"We have one minute left of our group time and then it will be time to go." Parent and child are free to clean up any toys or materials or leave them. They are not asked or required to clean up after the group time is over.

Give Form to Parents

As the parent and child leave the playroom, the professional should give each parent the Session Overview Form. This form should have been completed prior to the group meeting and provides the parents with information about what was addressed in the group meeting and information about the next weeks parent hosted playdate.

Goodbye Ritual

Establishing a goodbye ritual is optional in AutPlay play groups but professionals may want to consider the process. The goodbye ritual should be simple and the same one should be used to end each group meeting. This could be as simple as giving a high five to each child and parent as they leave the playroom or waving and saying "bye" to each child as they leave the room. The professional can create their own unique goodbye ritual but should remember to keep it simple and be consistent in using the same process at the end of each group meeting.

Play Group Session Two

Length

Based on a 50-minute group session.

About This Week's Group

The professional should take note of any specific information they want to cover or address in this group session. The professional should review and prep for the session time. Are there any specific toys or materials that need to be highlighted? Does the room need any adjustments? Is the Session Overview Form for parents completed and ready to give to parents? Remember that parents will remain in the waiting room until they join the group with about 20 minutes left.

The Table

Utilizing the "Table" concept is optional and may not be done in each session but should be considered as another tool to help promote social play. Possible toys for the table in session two might be Duplo Legos and/ or building blocks.

Structuring Statement

The professional begins the group with a simple structuring statement— "This is the playroom and you can play with anything you want in here, and I (we) will be in here with you." Nothing else needs to be said or explained to the children at this time.

Play and Social Time

The children will have 35 minutes of unstructured play time. They may play with anything they want, and the professional(s) will move around the playroom making tracking and reflective statements and trying to encourage interactive play with themselves and other children in the group. Tracking and reflective statements resemble those in Child Centered Play Therapy (Landreth, 1991). A tracking statement is tracking what the child is doing such as "You are scooping sand into the bucket," or "You are finished with the blocks and now you're playing with the cash register." Reflective statements reflect any emotion the child verbalizes or displays such as "You are frustrated you can't get that lid off," or "You like putting your hands in the sand," or "That makes you mad." The professional should try to make tracking and reflective states periodically for each of the children in the group.

Parent and Child Play Time

Parents join the group for the last 20 minutes. Once the parents are in the playroom, they are given the following directive: "This is your time to play and interact with your child or any other parent and child, and we will be in here with you." This is an opportunity for the professional to further observe the parent/child interaction, role model play attempts with the child, and allow for more social play experiences. The professional can roam around the playroom and attempt to get involved with any of the parents and children's play time. The professional may even want to role model or help some parents as they attempt to play with their children. The professional can also encourage group play among the parents and children.

Five Minute Warning

When there is around five minutes left of the group time, the professional will make the following statement "We have five minutes left of our group time today, then it will be time to go." The professional makes another statement when there is one minute left of group time—"We have one minute left of our group time and then it will be time to go." Parent and child are free to clean up any toys or materials or leave them. They are not asked or required to clean up after the group time is over.

Give Form to Parents

As the parent and child leave the playroom, the professional should give each parent the Session Overview Form. This form should have been completed prior to the group meeting and provides the parents with information about what was addressed in the group meeting and information about the next weeks parent hosted playdate.

Goodbye Ritual

If a goodbye ritual was created and started in session one, it should be continued in session two. If one was not started in session one, it can be started in session two. Remember to keep the goodbye ritual simple and consistent. An example might be to have each child line up at the door and as each child leaves, the professional gives them a fist pump.

Play Group Session Three

Length

Based on a 50-minute group session.

About This Week's Group

The professional should take note of any specific information they want to cover or address in this group session. The professional should review and prep for the session time. Are there any specific toys or materials that need to be highlighted? Does the room need any adjustments? Is the Session Overview Form for parents completed and ready to give to parents?

The Table

Utilizing the "Table" concept is optional and may not be done in each session but should be considered as another tool to help promote social play. Possible toys for the table in session three might be a couple of puzzles to put together (puzzles appropriate for the age and ability level of the group members).

Structuring Statement

The professional begins the group with a simple structuring statement— "This is the playroom and you can play with anything you want in here, and I (we) will be in here with you." Nothing else needs to be said or explained to the children at this time.

Play and Social Time

The children will have 35 minutes of unstructured play time. They may play with anything they want, and the professional(s) will move around the playroom making tracking and reflective statements and trying to encourage interactive play with themselves and other children in the group. Encouraging interactive play resembles the process of the Follow Me Approach in AutPlay Therapy (Grant, 2017). The professional periodically tries to get involved with what the child is playing. For example, if the child is playing in the sand tray, the professional will move beside the child and try to participate with the child and encourage interactive or reciprocal play. In AutPlay play groups, the professional can also try to involve other children in the reciprocal play. The professional should attempt to engage with each child in the group periodically but not force interactive play.

Parent and Child Play Time

Parents join the group for the last 20 minutes. Once the parents are in the playroom, they are given the following directive "This is your time to play and interact with your child or any other parent and child, and we will be in here with you." This is an opportunity for the professional to further observe the parent/child interaction, role model play attempts with the child, and allow for more social play experiences. It is likely that parents may have questions for the professional during this time. This is appropriate to a minimal degree and as questions relate directly to play times with their child or something happening in the moment. Other questions should be addressed at a different time so the parent and child play time can be exclusively focused on the parents playing with or attempting to play with their child.

Five Minute Warning

When there is around five minutes left of the group time, the professional will make the following statement: "We have five minutes left of our group time today, then it will be time to go." The professional makes another statement when there is one minute left of group time—"We have one minute left of our group time and then it will be time to go." Parent and child are free to clean up any toys or materials or leave them. They are not asked or required to clean up after the group time is over.

Give Form to Parents

Give each parent the completed Session Overview Form as they leave the playroom.

Goodbye Ritual

If a goodbye ritual has been established, it should be implemented. Remember, the same goodbye ritual should be used to end each group meeting.

Play Group Session Four

Length

Based on a 50-minute group session.

About This Week's Group

The professional should take note of any specific information they want to cover or address in this group session. The professional should review and prep for the session time. Are there any specific toys or materials that need to be highlighted? Does the room need any adjustments? Is the Session Overview Form for parents completed and ready to give to parents?

The Table

Utilizing the "Table" concept is optional and may not be done in each session but should be considered as another tool to help promote social play. Possible toys for the table in session four might be a large piece of white paper and crayons.

Structuring Statement

The professional begins the group with a simple structuring statement— "This is the playroom and you can play with anything you want in here, and I (we) will be in here with you." Nothing else needs to be said or explained to the children at this time.

Play and Social Time

The children will have 35 minutes of unstructured play time. They may play with anything they want, and the professional(s) will move around the playroom making tracking and reflective statements and trying to encourage interactive play with themselves and other children in the group.

Parent and Child Play Time

Parents join the group for the last 20 minutes. Once the parents are in the playroom, they are given the following directive: "This is your time to play and interact with your child or any other parent and child, and we will be in here with you." This is an opportunity for the professional to further observe the parent/child interaction, role model play attempts with the child, and allow for more social play experiences. The professional should continue to support each parent and child in their playtime.

Some parents may struggle with engaging with their child. The professional should be encouraging and supportive and assist any parents who may need help.

Five Minute Warning

When there is around five minutes left of the group time, the professional will make the following statement: "We have five minutes left of our group time today, then it will be time to go." The professional makes another statement when there is one minute left of group time—"We have one minute left of our group time and then it will be time to go." Parent and child are free to clean up any toys or materials or leave them. They are not asked or required to clean up after the group time is over.

Give Form to Parents

Give each parent the completed Session Overview Form as they leave the playroom.

Goodbye Ritual

If a goodbye ritual has been established, it should be implemented. Remember, the same goodbye ritual should be used to end each group meeting.

Play Group Session Five

Length

Based on a 50-minute group session.

About This Week's Group

The professional should take note of any specific information they want to cover or address in this group session. The professional should review and prep for the session time. Are there any specific toys or materials that need to be highlighted? Does the room need any adjustments? Is the Session Overview Form for parents completed and ready to give to parents? At this point, about half of the group process has been completed. Professionals might consider a having a short meeting with parents to evaluate how the process has been going for them. This meeting could be part of the group time or scheduled for a different time.

The Table

Utilizing the "Table" concept is optional and may not be done in each session but should be considered as another tool to help promote social play. Possible toys for the table in session five might be a train track or race car track.

Structuring Statement

The professional begins the group with a simple structuring statement— "This is the playroom and you can play with anything you want in here, and I (we) will be in here with you." Nothing else needs to be said or explained to the children at this time.

Play and Social Time

The children will have 35 minutes of unstructured play time. They may play with anything they want, and the professional(s) will move around the playroom making tracking and reflective statements and trying to encourage interactive play with themselves and other children in the group. This group meeting would be the halfway point in completing the group. The professional should take note of any progress made toward interactive play and continue to encourage this with the group members. For those children who have started to play more socially and reciprocally, the professional will want to encourage this play to continue with other children. The professional may want to focus more of their interactive play efforts on those children who are still lacking progress in this area.

Parent and Child Play Time

Parents join the group for the last 20 minutes. Once the parents are in the playroom, they are given the following directive: "This is your time to play and interact with your child or any other parent and child and we will be in here with you." This is the half-way portion of the group meetings. The professional should take note of the parent and child interactions and play of each member in the group and assess progress. Moving forward, the professional should focus more on those parents and children who are continuing to struggle with having an interactive play time.

Five Minute Warning

When there is around five minutes left of the group time, the professional will make the following statement: "We have five minutes left of our group time today, then it will be time to go." The professional makes another statement when there is one minute left of group time "We have one minute left of our group time and then it will be time to go." Parent and child are free to clean up any toys or materials or leave them. They are not asked or required to clean up after the group time is over.

Give Form to Parents

Give each parent the completed Session Overview Form as they leave the playroom.

Goodbye Ritual

If a goodbye ritual has been established, it should be implemented. Remember, the same goodbye ritual should be used to end each group meeting.

Play Group Session Six

Length

Based on a 50-minute group session.

About This Week's Group

The professional should take note of any specific information they want to cover or address in this group session. The professional should review and prep for the session time. Are there any specific toys or materials that need to be highlighted? Does the room need any adjustments? Is the Session Overview Form for parents completed and ready to give to parents? At this point, the professional will want to critically evaluate the children in the group in terms of how their social play seems to be improving or is still lacking. The professional may want to target children more specifically in encouraging social play.

The Table

Utilizing the "Table" concept is optional and may not be done in each session but should be considered as another tool to help promote social play. Possible toys for the table in session six might be Mr. and Mrs. Potato Head.

Structuring Statement

The professional begins the group with a simple structuring statement— "This is the playroom and you can play with anything you want in here, and I (we) will be in here with you." Nothing else needs to be said or explained to the children at this time.

Play and Social Time

The children will have 35 minutes of unstructured play time. They may play with anything they want, and the professional(s) will move around the playroom making tracking and reflective statements and trying to encourage interactive play with themselves and other children in the group. Interactive play attempts should be focused on the children who are most lacking this type of social play skill.

Parent and Child Play Time

Parents join the group for the last 20 minutes. Once the parents are in the playroom, they are given the following directive: "This is your time to play and interact with your child or any other parent and child and we will be in here with you." This is an opportunity for the professional to assist parents in having a positive and interactive play time with their child.

Five Minute Warning

When there is around five minutes left of the group time, the professional will make the following statement: "We have five minutes left of our group time today, then it will be time to go." The professional makes another statement when there is one minute left of group time—"We have one minute left of our group time and then it will be time to go." Parent and child are free to clean up any toys or materials or leave them. They are not asked or required to clean up after the group time is over.

Give Form to Parents

Give each parent the completed Session Overview Form as they leave the playroom.

Goodbye Ritual

If a goodbye ritual has been established, it should be implemented. Remember, the same goodbye ritual should be used to end each group meeting.

Play Group Session Seven

Length

Based on a 50-minute group session.

About This Week's Group

The professional should take note of any specific information they want to cover or address in this group session. The professional should review and prep for the session time. Are there any specific toys or materials that need to be highlighted? Does the room need any adjustments? Is the Session Overview Form for parents completed and ready to give to parents?

The Table

Utilizing the "Table" concept is optional and may not be done in each session but should be considered as another tool to help promote social play. Possible toys for the table in session seven might be a few board games or card games (age and functioning ability appropriate).

Structuring Statement

The professional begins the group with a simple structuring statement— "This is the playroom and you can play with anything you want in here, and I (we) will be in here with you." Nothing else needs to be said or explained to the children at this time.

Play and Social Time

The children will have 35 minutes of unstructured play time. They may play with anything they want, and the professional(s) will move around the playroom making tracking and reflective statements and trying to encourage interactive play with themselves and other children in the group. Interactive play attempts should be focused on the children who are most lacking this type of social play skill.

Parent and Child Play Time

Parents join the group for the last 20 minutes. Once the parents are in the playroom, they are given the following directive "This is your time to play and interact with your child or any other parent and child, and we will be in here with you." This is an opportunity for the professional to assist parents in having a positive and interactive play time with their child.

Five Minute Warning

When there is around five minutes left of the group time, the professional will make the following statement: "We have five minutes left of our group time today, then it will be time to go." The professional makes another statement when there is one minute left of group time—"We have one minute left of our group time and then it will be time to go." Parent and child are free to clean up any toys or materials or leave them. They are not asked or required to clean up after the group time is over.

Give Form to Parents

Give each parent the completed Session Overview Form as they leave the playroom.

Goodbye Ritual

If a goodbye ritual has been established, it should be implemented. Remember, the same goodbye ritual should be used to end each group meeting.

Play Group Session Eight

Length

Based on a 50-minute group session.

About This Week's Group

The professional should take note of any specific information they want to cover or address in this group session. The professional should review and prep for the session time. Are there any specific toys or materials that need to be highlighted? Does the room need any adjustments? Is the Session Overview Form for parents completed and ready to give to parents?

The Table

Utilizing the "Table" concept is optional and may not be done in each session but should be considered as another tool to help promote social play. Possible toys for the table in session eight might be a bowling set or ring toss game.

Structuring Statement

The professional begins the group with a simple structuring statement—"This is the playroom and you can play with anything you want in here, and I (we) will be in here with you." Nothing else needs to be said or explained to the children at this time.

Play and Social Time

The children will have 35 minutes of unstructured play time. They may play with anything they want, and the professional(s) will move around the playroom making tracking and reflective statements and trying to encourage interactive play with themselves and other children in the group. Interactive play attempts should be focused on the children who are most lacking this type of social play skill.

Parent and Child Play Time

Parents join the group for the last 20 minutes. Once the parents are in the playroom, they are given the following directive: "This is your time to play and interact with your child or any other parent and child and we will be in here with you." This is an opportunity for the professional to assist parents in having a positive and interactive play time with their child.

Five Minute Warning

When there is around five minutes left of the group time, the professional will make the following statement: "We have five minutes left of our group time today, then it will be time to go." The professional makes another statement when there is one minute left of group time—"We have one minute left of our group time and then it will be time to go." Parent and child are free to clean up any toys or materials or leave them. They are not asked or required to clean up after the group time is over.

Give Form to Parents

Give each parent the completed Session Overview Form as they leave the playroom.

Goodbye Ritual

If a goodbye ritual has been established, it should be implemented. Remember, the same goodbye ritual should be used to end each group meeting.

Play Group Session Nine

Length

Based on a 50-minute group session.

About This Week's Group

The professional should take note of any specific information they want to cover or address in this group session. The professional should review and prep for the session time. Are there any specific toys or materials that need to be highlighted? Does the room need any adjustments? Is the Session Overview Form for parents completed and ready to give to parents?

The Table

Utilizing the "Table" concept is optional and may not be done in each session but should be considered as another tool to help promote social play. Possible toys for the table in session nine might be puppets.

Structuring Statement

The professional begins the group with a simple structuring statement—"This is the playroom and you can play with anything you want in here, and I (we) will be in here with you." Nothing else needs to be said or explained to the children at this time.

Play and Social Time

The children will have 35 minutes of unstructured play time. They may play with anything they want, and the professional(s) will move around the playroom making tracking and reflective statements and trying to encourage interactive play with themselves and other children in the group. Interactive play attempts should be focused on the children who are most lacking this type of social play skill.

Parent and Child Play Time

Parents join the group for the last 20 minutes. Once the parents are in the playroom, they are given the following directive "This is your time to play and interact with your child or any other parent and child, and we will be in here with you." This is an opportunity for the professional to assist parents in having a positive and interactive play time with their child. The professional should note that there is only one group meeting left after this one. If the professional feels it is necessary, he or she could meet individually with any parent and child who may still be struggling and could benefit from a more focused session with the professional to work on joint play skills.

Five Minute Warning

When there is around five minutes left of the group time, the professional will make the following statement: "We have five minutes left of our group time today, then it will be time to go." The professional makes another statement when there is one minute left of group time—"We have one minute left of our group time and then it will be time to go." Parent and child are free to clean up any toys or materials or leave them. They are not asked or required to clean up after the group time is over.

Give Form to Parents

Give each parent the completed Session Overview Form as they leave the playroom.

Goodbye Ritual

If a goodbye ritual has been established, it should be implemented. Remember, the same goodbye ritual should be used to end each group meeting.

Play Group Session Ten

Length

Based on a 50-minute group session.

About This Week's Group

The professional should take note of any specific information they want to cover or address in this group session. The professional should review and prep for the session time. Are there any specific toys or materials that need to be highlighted? Does the room need any adjustments? Is the Session Overview Form for parents completed and ready to give to parents? This is the final in clinic group meeting. The professional may want to have a short meeting with each parent to discuss participation in future groups or possibly continuing with the play group. AutPlay play groups can be ongoing and this is often encouraged as children with autism typically benefit from more than 10 sessions.

The Table

Utilizing the "Table" concept is optional and may not be done in each session but should be considered as another toll to help promote social play. Possible toys for the table in session ten might be a sand tray and sand tray toys.

Structuring Statement

The professional begins the group with a simple structuring statement— "This is the playroom and you can play with anything you want in here, and I (we) will be in here with you." The professional should mention to the children that this will be the last group meeting.

Play and Social Time

This is the last play group meeting and the professional should continue with the same process as he or she has been implementing. The play time length might be shortened to around 25 minutes to provide more time for a final goodbye ritual and any closure processes that need to be implemented. They children will continue to play with anything they want, and the professional(s) will move around the playroom making tracking and reflective statements and trying to encourage interactive play with themselves and other children in the group. Interactive play attempts should be focused on the children who are most lacking this type of social play skill.

Parent and Child Play Time

This is the last session and the parent and child play time proceeds as usually with the parents joining the group for the last 20 minutes. The professional may want to shorten the parent and child play time to have more time for the final goodbye ritual and to discuss any closure issues with the parents. This would also be an appropriate time to discuss moving forward with continuing the group, starting a new group, or working individually with some of the parents and children.

Five Minute Warning

When there is around five minutes left of the group time, the professional will make the following statement: "We have five minutes left of our group time today, then it will be time to go." The professional makes another statement when there is one minute left of group time—"We have one minute left of our group time and then it will be time to go." Parent and child are free to clean up any toys or materials or leave them. They are not asked or required to clean up after the group time is over.

Give Form to Parents

Give each parent the completed Session Overview Form as they leave the playroom. This is the last session, and this should be noted on the form. There is technically one more parent-hosted play date scheduled for the next week—this should be noted on the form. Parents are encouraged to continue having play dates with the other children and parents as they wish.

Goodbye Ritual

Since this is the last group session. The professional may want to take more time and express a goodbye and thank you for playing in the group to the children and allow them to express a goodbye to the other children if they would like. The professional should have prepared, and give to each parent and child, a certificate of completion. A sample certificate of completion is provided in the appendix section of this book. If it has been established that the group will continue to meet, then the standard goodbye ritual can be implemented.

6 AutPlay® Therapy Social Skills Groups (10-Session Model)

Social skills groups are an intervention strategy in which two or more children diagnosed with ASD or a related condition come together and are simultaneously taught a variety of social behaviors. These groups have been found to be effective in teaching a wide variety of behaviors, including social interaction, greetings, handling disagreements, sportsmanship, and managing emotions. There are many potential benefits for implementing social skills groups for children diagnosed with ASD; these benefits include possible increased observational learning by placing peers in closer proximity to each other and increasing the likelihood of generalization of skills outside the social skills group (Leaf et al., 2017).

AutPlay social skill groups are based off the AutPlay Therapy directive interventions phase of treatment. In this phase of treatment, the child and parent are both present during the sessions and taught directive play therapy interventions which are practiced during session times. The professional teaches the parent how to continue to implement the interventions at home between sessions. This process continues until treatment goals are meet. AutPlay Therapy directive play therapy interventions are specifically designed to meet a child where they are in terms of their level of skill development. AutPlay Therapy directive play therapy interventions are designed to help increase play skills, social skills, and other needed abilities such as emotional regulation skills. AutPlay Therapy takes into account the lack of play skills that may be present in a child with ASD and introduces play in a directive and specific manner so that children with an ASD can participate and learn from the play-based interventions.

AutPlay social skills groups mimic the directive interventions phase in AutPlay therapy. In each clinic meeting, the group participants are taught a specific social skill using directive play therapy interventions designed to help improve social skill deficits. Parents are then encouraged to support the interventions and skills being address at home between group meetings. Parents are also taught how to host a meeting with the group participants outside of the clinical setting. This is an opportunity for the participants to have a less formal gathering to practice being social with each other. Incorporating parent involvement and the utilization of directive play therapy interventions are both processes in AutPlay social skills groups taken directly from AutPlay Therapy protocol.

Pragmatics of AutPlay Therapy Social Skills Groups

Definition of AutPlay Therapy Social Skills Groups—These groups focus on improving social functioning and are designed for elementary, middle, and high school aged children who have been diagnosed with autism or a related condition. Children and adolescents who do not have a diagnosis but struggle with social skill challenges can also participate. The functioning level of the child does not matter but they must be able to participate on some level in directive interventions—otherwise, participating in an AutPlay play group would be more appropriate.

Role of the Professional—The professional organizes and facilitates the AutPlay social skills group process. The professional is a player and an encourager for both the children and the parents. Often, the professional also serves as a role model and instructor. The professional is active in the social skills groups by teaching specific social skill play interventions, establishing limits when necessary, and providing support and strategies to parents.

Structure—AutPlay social skill groups are typically 20 group sessions each lasting around one hour. The group begins with a meeting in the professional's clinic where social skills are taught and practiced though various play therapy interventions. The next week, the group participants meet together outside of the clinic to have a less formal "hang out" time. This meeting is hosted by one of the participant's parents. The meetings alternate in this fashion week to week for 20 meetings—10 in clinic skills training sessions and 10 outside "hang out" meetings. A step-by-step organization and structure guide for starting an AutPlay social skills group is provided in the appendix section of this book.

Generating Interest in a Group—Professionals should assess in their local community the need for social skills groups. This can be done by contacting local agencies that work with children and adolescents with ASD, contacting school programs, and checking with local parent support groups.

Organization of a Group—The professional should decide on a possible start date and location for the group. The professional should also prepare any forms needed for the group and begin to market the group. A sample marketing flier is provided in the appendix section of this book.

Assessing/Screening Group Members—It is important that group members are as similar as possible when it comes to age and developmental level. Gender tends to not be as important as having children in the same group who are around the same functioning level. When you have groups with many ages and several different functioning levels, you lose some of the environmental conditions that help develop social skills. The Intake Form and Group Readiness Questionnaire found in the appendix section of this book can be used to help assess group participants.

The professional should meet with each parent and child who might be interested in participating in a social skills group. This meeting is an opportunity to complete necessary paperwork, assess the child's ability level, and decide if the child would be an appropriate fit for the group that is beginning. If the child is assessed to not be ready for a group experience, the professional should try to offer meeting with the child for individual therapy and working toward joining a group. The professional can offer more than one group. This might be especially helpful if there are different ages and developmental levels wanting to attend—the professional could offer multiple groups, matching the children with the best fit group. It might be necessary to place some children on a group wait list until there are enough children interested in participating in a group that are at the same age and developmental level.

> *Who Can Participate*—Any child or adolescent can participate in an AutPlay social skills group. Participants do not need a formal diagnosis of ASD. Although a primary focus of the group is autism issues, any child who might benefit from the social skill work of the group could participate.
>
> *Group Size*—The typical size of a group should be four to six children, with no more than eight. Anything larger will negatively affect the ability of the group to naturally connect and work on social skills. Groups can be smaller and still be beneficial, but larger groups should be avoided. It would likely be better to have two groups of four than one group of eight. The minimum number of participants for a group is two. Professionals should strive for a ratio of one adult for every two children, so the larger the group size, the more adults that will be needed to facilitate the group. These are recommendations for group size. This will vary depending on the age and functioning level of the participants. It might be possible for one professional to work with a group of four children if they were older children and their functioning ability was high.
>
> *Length of Group Meetings*—The length of time a group meets may vary depending on the professional's preference, but the group structure for AutPlay social skills groups is based on a one-hour group session. Some professionals may prefer to lengthen the group time.

Number of Group Meetings—AutPlay social skills groups meet for 10 in clinic formal teaching times and 10 outside of the clinic less formal "hang out" times. There is a total of 20 meetings. The formal and informal meetings alternate week to week. The first week the group meets in the clinic, the next week they meet outside of the clinic. The professional does not attend the outside-the-clinic meeting; this is hosted by one of the participant's parents. The professional can begin new groups at any time or start another group when one ends, and the new groups can include some of the same participants from a previous group. It is important to formally end a group after the 20 meetings to give children a clean opportunity to leave the group.

Play Development—Since much of the group focus will be on participating in play therapy interventions, it is important to assess each child's play skills and deficits. The AutPlay Groups Assessment of Play Form is provided in the appendix section of this book. The professional will give the parent the play assessment to complete as part of the group intake process prior to the group beginning.

Social Skill Development—AutPlay social skills groups provide an integrative process of clinical and natural opportunity for children and adolescents to develop social skills. A formal, more directive social skills training happens during the in-clinic meetings while a less formal, more naturalist process happens outside of the clinic meetings. Both experiences are important for children with autism to gain social skills.

Group Meeting Locations—The professional will likely have in-clinic meetings at his or her clinic or some arranged meeting place. It is ideal for the in-clinic meeting location to stay consistent throughout the duration of the group. For the parent-hosted, outside-the-clinic meetings, there are many options where a group could meet (this is typically decided on by the parent who is hosting). A common setting, such as a parent's home, a church, or a support group meeting facility, would certainly work. It is highly encouraged that some of the social group meetings occur in public. This may be a certain event, or specific activity designed for children; it may simply be going to a restaurant or park. Some parents may need help in deciding where to meet. Table 6.1 provides some meeting place options for parents. Also, the professional should communicate to parents that the parent-hosted meetings should not include any formal social skills interventions. This is a time for the participants to be together and practice natural socialization. The parents can help their child to interact and practice skills they have been working on but there should be no pressure or purposeful teaching. The participants need this time to be with other children and enjoy a group experience.

Table 6.1 Meeting Places for Parent-Hosted Social Skills Groups

Arcade	Nature Center
Botanical Garden	Area Lake
Special Events (Art Fest, Cider Days, Autism Fairs)	Zoo
YMCA/Community Center	Public Pool
Discovery Center	Various Stores
Restaurants	Movie Theater
Entertainment Center	Jump House
Sporting Event	Museum
Farms	Fair/Carnival/Circus
Amusement Park	Miniature Golf
Go Carts	Fishing/Canoeing/Hiking
Picnic	Public Library
Pottery Studio	Farmers Market
State Parks	Imax
Ice Skating Rink/Roller Skating	Road Trip
Neighborhood Walk	Mall
Church Events	Grocery Store
Pumpkin Patch	Post Office
Horse Stables	Animal Shelter

It is helpful for parents to understand the dynamics of the children in the group and where each child is at in terms of functioning level and tolerance for certain situations such as any sensory issues or fears related to certain environments. Any information about any of the group participants that would guide the selection of location or event for a parent-hosted meeting should be shared with the parents to avoid any potential issues. Where to meet and the type of hang out experience should be decided on and communicated the week before the parent-hosted meeting. Typically, the professional will have this information and share it with all the children and parents at the end of the in-clinic meeting. This information is included on the Session Overview Form (located in the appendix section) that is given to the parents at the end of each in-clinic meeting.

   Handling Unwanted Behavior—The professional will want to choose one of the limit setting models defined in this book and explain the limit setting model to the participants during the first meeting. The professional should use the limit setting model consistently. Each model provides for a final consequence of ending the group time for the child if the behavior does not change and/or is too disruptive. The professional should be patient and implement limits at a minimum. It is expected that there will be some unwanted and troublesome behavior. If it is something the professional can work with and correct easily, then there is no need for further consequence. If possible, the professional should establish a break room or area that the participants can go to if they are needing a break. This is something the professional can lead the child to or the child can initiate a break themselves. If a break room is established, the professional should explain this to the participants during the first session.

When parents are hosting a group meeting, the professional will not typically be present. The parents may need a brief instruction on how to handle unwanted behavior. This is more fully explained in Chapter 4. It's important to explain to parents that behaviors will likely occur during a parent-hosted meeting. If a parent has certain strategies they typically implement to help their child calm, the parent should implement these strategies. If a parent feels like they need to leave the meeting this is okay. The parent and child should leave, and they can try again at the next meeting. Other parents should get involved only if the parent of the child with unwanted behavior asks for assistance. It is important that the parent of the child having the unwanted behavior is the primary person addressing their child and trying to manage the behavior.

Parents as Co-Change Agents—Parents participate in the AutPlay social skills groups. In AutPlay Therapy, parents work with the professional in learning interventions to help their child gain skills. In AutPlay social skills groups, parents host a group meeting outside of the clinic to help further the acquisition of social skill gains. This process is fully explained to parents during the initial consultation about the social skills group. Any training, suggestions, or help a parent may need should be provided by the professional. If a parent has concerns and would like suggestions for hosting a group time, the professional should meet with the parent and provide the information they are requesting. The professional should communicate to parents that they are an important part of the group process and empower parents to feel confident in their participation.

When parents host a group meeting, other parents should participate in each group meeting as much as possible. It may not be necessary for every parent to be at every meeting if parents are comfortable with others taking care of their children (this will depend on the size of the group and the developmental and functioning level of group participants). It is important that there are enough parents at each group meeting to care for the children and facilitate the group. Social groups provide a good opportunity for parents to socialize and find support, thus is it recommended that parents participate with their children as often as they can.

10-SESSION GUIDE FOR IN CLINIC AUTPLAY SOCIAL SKILLS GROUPS

Note: Professionals should review the step-by-step guide for beginning an AutPlay group. This is located in the appendix section of this book.

Social Skills Group Session One

Length

Based on a one-hour group session.

About this week's group

The professional should take note of any specific information they want to cover or address in this group session. The professional should review and prep for the session time. Are there any materials needed for the intervention? Does the therapist have an icebreaker and closing activity planned? Is the Session Overview Form for parents completed and ready to give to parents?

Welcome icebreaker

Welcome the participants and ask each participant to share their name and something they like doing. It can be a video game, a sport, any activity. Each professional should go first, introducing themselves and role modeling how to share as well as what information to share. This should be brief, only taking about 10 minutes.

First session information

In the first session only, the professional will want to briefly go over the structure of the group sessions, what the participants can expect each week, and how the parent hosted outside of the clinic meetings work. The professional will also want to cover any group rules such as being positive with each other. The professional will also want to cover the limit setting model that will be used to address any limits that need to be set. If there is a process for participants to take a break if they are feeling dysregulated, this process should be explained to the group participants.

Anything to share

This will be an active part of each group session where the participants will have an opportunity to share anything they would like with the group. In the first session it is likely there will not be much sharing, but this will increase as the group meets more often. The anything to share time gives the group participants an opportunity to get to know each other better, practice their speaking and listening skills, and engage in reciprocal conversation. Professionals should monitor for any limit setting that is needed such as limiting the length of time someone talks, subject matter, and negative responses.

Implement the social skills intervention

A sample intervention for children (elementary age) and adolescents (middle and high school age) is provided. The professional is welcome to use the social skills interventions in this book and implement them in any order which they feel is appropriate. The professional can also use their own social skills interventions which they have created or acquired from other sources.

Process and application of the intervention

The professional will want to allow for some processing and application of the social skills intervention. An example of processing and application is provided at the end of each social skill intervention description.

Goodbye ritual

The professional should end each session with a goodbye ritual. This can change session to session, or the professional can repeat the same goodbye ritual each time. An example would be creating a special group handshake that each participant does to each other as they leave the group. This should be brief only taking about five minutes.

Give form to parents

As the children leave the group session, the professional should give each parent the Session Overview Form. Professionals will want to have the form completed prior to the group session.

GROUP SESSION ONE EXAMPLE SOCIAL SKILLS INTERVENTION FOR CHILDREN

Activity: Quiet and Loud

Social Skill Target Area(s)

Appropriate voice levels (speaking)

Level

Children

Materials Needed

None

Introduction

Quiet and Loud provides the opportunity for children to practice their speaking levels and tone of voice in a playful and engaging manner. Often children with autism and developmental disorders struggle with speaking too loudly, too softly, or in a monotone voice without appropriate inflection. This intervention is designed to help improve skill deficits in recognizing how the voice can fluctuate and how the child can control the tone and fluctuation.

Instructions

1. The professional tells the child they are going to complete an activity that works on how the child speaks and how their voice can be quiet, loud, or in between.
2. The professional demonstrates for the child by pressing their hands together in front of them and begins by saying something in a whisper. The professional moves their hands apart slowly, and progressively keeps moving their hands further apart. While the professional is continually moving their hands further apart, the professional is increasing the loudness of their voice.
3. The professional then asks the children to complete the process the professional just demonstrated. They will complete it as a group with the professional.
4. The professional then asks the children to complete the activity with a partner. The children can pick a word to say and that is the word they will use to go from a quiet to loud voice.

5. The professional asks the children to notice when they think their voice is too quiet and when it is too loud.
6. The professional then asks the children to do the intervention while trying to change the tone of their voice to match an emotion such as being sad, being scared, being excited, or being angry.

Processing and Application

The professional discusses with the children places and situations where it would be appropriate to talk in a whisper, normal voice, or loudly such as in a library, at home, or at a sporting event. This intervention works on increasing social skills, especially related to speaking in an appropriate volume for the situation and how to fluctuate tone of voice to mirror various feelings and states that the child may be experiencing. It is likely that this intervention will need to be played multiple times to help the child gain mastery and increase their speaking and tone skills.

GROUP SESSION ONE EXAMPLE SOCIAL SKILLS INTERVENTION FOR ADOLESCENTS

Activity: Divide and Conquer

Social Skill Target Area(s)

Connection, engagement, and teamwork

Level

Adolescents

Materials Needed

Balloons

Introduction

Adolescents with autism and other developmental disorders often have challenges in working with others and participating as part of a team. This intervention focuses on helping adolescents to notice others and work with another person to accomplish a task. It incorporates a teamwork concept in a fun and engaging game format.

Instructions

1. The professional explains to the group that they are going to play a game where the focus is on working together as a team.
2. The professional divides the group into pairs and each pair chooses an area to stand in the room.
3. The professional explains to the group that they can position themselves and their feet anywhere in the room but once in place, they have to pretend that their feet are stuck to the floor and cannot be moved.
4. The adolescent and their partner hit a balloon in the air back and forth and try to keep it from touching the ground without moving their feet.
5. The professional should spend some time discussing with the group the concept of working together and teamwork and that the only way to succeed at the game is by paying attention to each other and working as a team.
6. The group participants can also strategize and develop a plan deciding where each person will stand to cover the most room space.

7. If the balloon hits the ground, the pair can decide on a different place to stand and start over seeing if they can keep the balloon in the air longer. The game can be started over and played multiple times.

Processing and Application

The professional should process and ask the group what it felt like to work with another person, what felt easy and what felt hard? The professional can also ask participants to share about real life experiences where they had to work as part of a team or with another person to accomplish something. This intervention promotes body awareness skills, personal space, and self-control. Participants must work together to keep the balloon from hitting the ground, communicate to coordinate where they are going to stand to try and cover as much space as possible in the room, and often readjust and discuss how they are going to keep the balloon from touching the ground.

Social Skills Group Session Two

Length

Based on a one-hour group session.

About this week's group

The professional should continue to take note of any specific information they want to cover in this group session, as well as review and prep for the session. Prep would include having a list of statements ready for the icebreaker activity, having a general joy or sorrow ready to share, and finding a goodbye poem for the ending ritual. Materials for this session should be created and displayed. The icebreaker and closing activity should be practiced and the Session Overview Form ready to give to parents.

Welcome icebreaker

That's Like Me icebreaker carries over from session one in which clients are able to share something about themselves. The professional begins by stating something about his or herself (example: "I love winter"). Any group member who agrees with this statement calls out "That's Like Me." Each group member can then share a statement about themselves, and other group members can state "That's Like Me" when they agree with the statement. The professional should be prepared to prompt members with ideas if needed (examples include favorite season, favorite food, worst school subject, members in family, etc.). The icebreaker should take five to ten minutes maximum.

Anything to share

There may be more sharing during this group session, but there may also be some participants who are not ready. It may be helpful for the professional to ask the group members if they have any joys or sorrows to share from the past week and model an example if needed. The professional should keep their joy or sorrow general so as not to influence any group member's responses (example: "I had a great dinner last night," "I didn't have an umbrella on the rainy day last Thursday," etc.). The professional is an active listener at this time, and monitors for any limit setting needed.

Implement the social skills intervention

A sample intervention for children and adolescents is provided. The professional is welcome to use the social skills interventions in this book and implement them in any order which they feel is appropriate. The professional can also use their own social skills interventions which they have created or acquired from other sources.

Process and application of the intervention

The professional will want to allow for some processing and application of the social skills intervention. An example of processing and application is provided at the end of each social skill intervention description.

Goodbye ritual

The professional should end the session with the goodbye ritual from the previous session or create a new one for this session. An example would be reading a poem found online about saying goodbye.

Give form to parents

As the children leave the group session, the professional should give each parent the Session Overview Form. The professional will want to have the form completed prior to the group session.

GROUP SESSION TWO EXAMPLE SOCIAL SKILLS INTERVENTION FOR CHILDREN

Activity: Listen and Speak

Social Skill Target Area(s)

Listening without interrupting and sharing with others

Level

Children

Materials Needed

One mouth template glued onto a craft stick and enough ear templates glued onto craft sticks for each member of the group (the professional can draw and cut out mouth and ear pics or print off templates online). Multicolor crayons, or multiple shades of peach, brown, and black crayons, and a one-minute sand timer (can also use timer on cell phone, etc.).

Introduction

Listen and Speak is a fun way for children to practice speaking in a group as well as listening without interrupting. This can be a difficult skill, so the professional wants to keep it light and encouraging. The ear and mouth templates are a fun way to remind the members what their role is as the speaker or the listener. The professional does not expect any group member to speak for the entire minute, but encourages each child to attempt some verbalization, and does set a limit of one-minute speaking. The professional is also not expecting a continued conversation on the same subject matter; that is an advanced skill that is not necessary for this activity. Children can speak about whatever they want during their time.

Instructions

1. The professional tells the group that they are going to complete an activity that helps all of us learn how to listen better to others and how to speak about something they like.
2. The professional keeps the mouth prop and passes out one ear prop to each group member. Members are encouraged to color the ear if they like with the crayons provided.
3. The professional explains that in this game, whoever holds the mouth is the speaker. The speaker will turn over the sand timer, and then talk about whatever they want for one minute. They can talk less

than that, but not more than one minute. Those who hold the ear props are the listeners. The ears need to listen to the speaker and not interrupt.

4. The professional begins by holding the mouth prop up to their mouth and speaking for one minute. The group members hold the ear props up to one of their ears and listen.

5. When one minute is up, the professional congratulates the members on their hard work, and may need remind the members of expectations. The professional then passes the mouth to a group member and takes their ear prop. The activity is completed when every person has a turn as the speaker.

Processing and Application

The professional discusses with the group members the importance of using their voices to share with others, as well as listening to others without interrupting. The group discusses when these skills are important at home, school, and other environments. The professional makes sure each group member has the mouth and ear templates to take home for practice.

GROUP SESSION TWO EXAMPLE SOCIAL SKILLS INTERVENTION FOR ADOLESCENTS

Activity: Where I Stand

Social Skills Target Area(s)

Sharing with others, socializing with others, and understanding others' points of view

Level

Adolescents

Materials Needed

One long piece of yarn taped to the floor (yarn should be long enough to have all group members stand comfortably on the yarn with space between them). Two index cards taped to the floor on each end of the yarn. The word "YES!" should be written on one index card; "NO" on the other index card. A sample yes and no question is provided at the end of this activity description.

Introduction

Adolescents with autism are often rigid thinkers who see things in "black or white." This intervention helps them notice that other peers may not think or feel the same way they do. This intervention also allows group members to share and socialize in a structured format.

Instructions

1.   Before the group members arrive, the professional tapes a long piece of yarn to the floor and places the "YES!" index card at one end and the "NO!" index card at the other.
2.   The professional explains to the group that they are going to play a game to get to know each other better. The professional explains that they will say out loud a statement, and each group member should respond to the statement by standing on the yarn to the degree of how they feel about the statement. The closer they are to the "YES!" index card is the more they agree with the statement; the closer they are to the "NO!" index card is the more they disagree with the statement. The professional may need to check for understanding and give a few examples.

3. The professional says aloud the first statement and gives everyone time to choose where they are going to stand on the yarn. When everyone has chosen a place, the professional invites any group member to share why they chose where they stood on the line. The professional may also suggest that group members look around and notice how members feel differently about the question.
4. The professional continues this game until all statements are read.

Processing and Application

The professional is making sure during this activity that group members are being respectful of differing opinions. The group discusses what they learned about each other and themselves during the activity. Some questions the professional can ask include: Were you surprised about anything you learned? Were any of the statements difficult for you to decide where to stand? After listening to other group members, were you considering moving to a different spot on the yarn?

Sample Yes and No Statements

- I like to have people around me.
- I sleep well at night.
- I do well in school.
- I am honest.
- I do my homework.
- I play computer games.
- I am smart.
- I am a happy person.
- I eat healthy.
- I have friends.
- I help my siblings.
- I have meltdowns.
- I love to eat sweets.
- I play outside.
- I like to swim.
- I live with my mom and dad.
- I am funny.
- I wake up easily in the morning.
- My teacher likes me.
- I do my own laundry.
- I like to play sports.
- Math is my best subject.

Social Skills Group Session Three

Length

Based on a one-hour group session

About this week's group

The professional should continue to take note of any specific information they want to cover in this group session, as well as review and prep for the session. Prep would include having examples of ways to line up for the icebreaker, by having a general joy or sorrow ready to share and by having goodbye in different languages. Materials for this session should be created and displayed. The icebreaker and closing activity should be practiced and the Session Overview Form ready to give to parents.

Welcome icebreaker

Line Up is a short game which allows the group members to work together while discovering a bit more about each other. The professional calls out, "Everyone line up according to . . ." (examples include youngest to oldest, alphabetical older, shortest to tallest, etc.). Group members discover together how they all need to line up.

Anything to share

The professional should follow the same suggestions from group session one or two.

Implement the social skills intervention

The professional can use the interventions provided in the following, in the appendix of this book, or one of their own.

Process and application of the intervention

An example of processing and application is provided at the end of each social skill intervention description.

Goodbye ritual

Teach the group members ways to say goodbye in other languages and have them choose one goodbye they will say to others.

Spanish: Adios
French: Au Revoir

German: Auf Wiedersehen
Italian: Arrivederci
Japanese: Sayonara
Hindi: Namaste
Arabic: Ma'a as-salaama
Hawaiian: Aloha

Give form to parents

As the children leave the group session, the professional should give each parent the Session Overview Form. The professional will want to have the form completed prior to the group.

GROUP SESSION THREE EXAMPLE SOCIAL SKILLS INTERVENTION FOR CHILDREN

Activity: Space Please!

Social Skill Target Area

Identifying needs and social boundaries, understanding others' body language, understanding others' point of view, and expressing own opinion.

Level

Children

Materials Needed

Several pool noodles, some original size, some cut in half, some cut in quarters.

Introduction

Space Please! activity allows group members to determine how much personal space they need to feel comfortable. They will also discover others may need more or less personal space than they do. Often, children with autism believe that their comfort level mirrors others, and this can cause difficulty with peer relationships. Since it can be very hard to recognize the social cues of their peers, these children may not understand they are standing too close or too far away from someone. This activity will help students realize they may need to ask their peers if they are comfortable with where they are standing.

Instructions

1. Divide the group into pairs. If there is an odd number, the professional should be a group member.
2. Give each pair a full-sized pool noodle. Instruct each group member to place one end of the noodle on each of their stomachs and hold it there.
3. Keeping the pool noodle on each of their bellies, pairs should have a conversation. If the group members struggle with this, the professional could ask a general question to stimulate conversation.
4. When finished, have pairs drop the full-sized noodle and give each group member a half-sized pool noodle. Follow the same directions as with the full-sized pool noodle.

5. When finished, have pairs drop the half-sized pool noodle and give each group member a quarter-sized pool noodle. Follow the same directions as with the previous sized noodles.

Processing and Application

Once this activity has been completed, the group members should come together and sit in a circle with each other. The professional should ask each group member when they felt the most comfortable as far as personal space. Was one noodle-length too close, too far, just right? Point out after each participant shares the similarities and differences they shared. Discuss ways that group members could share with their parents, teachers, and peers the amount of personal space they need, as well as ways to decide if they are giving others enough personal space.

GROUP SESSION THREE EXAMPLE SOCIAL SKILLS INTERVENTION FOR ADOLESCENTS

Activity: Personal Space

Social Skill Target Area(s)

Identifying needs and social boundaries, understanding others' body language, understanding others' point of view, and expressing own opinion

Level

Adolescents

Materials Needed

Several balls of yarn and scissors

Introduction

This is an excellent way for clients to work on recognizing the body language and facial expressions of their peers. It can also help them see that everyone has different needs and that personal space is personal to all. Individuals with autism often have theory of mind deficits, and this intervention can help improve this skill.

Instructions

1. The professional discusses how we all need a certain amount of space between us to feel comfortable.
2. The professional models this activity with one of the group participants. The professional hands the child the end of the yarn, while the professional holds the ball of yarn.
3. The professional invites the participant to hold the yarn and walk all the way to one side of the room. The professional unrolls the yarn and walks to the other side of the room.
4. The professional and participant face each other from each side of the room. The professional explains that they will take one step forward then stop. Other members are to watch the body language of the participant and decide if the professional is too far away, close enough, or too close. The participant then shares if the group is correct based on how they are feeling.
5. If the professional is too far away (which hopefully is the case, so take a very small step!) they will then take another step, stop and ask

members to decide too far, close enough, too close. The participant then shares how they feel.

6. This continues until the group members or the participant says that the professional is close enough (where they will stop) or too close (where they will back up). Once the professional is at the close enough point, they will cut the string and give to the participant.

7. Participants can work in pairs to complete this activity as described earlier, until everyone has their own personal space yarn piece.

8. Discuss what was noticed in body language surrounding comfort and discomfort, the differences in personal space needs, etc.

9. Yarn can be brought home to help family and friends learn how much space is needed.

Processing and Application

Processing includes discussion on what group members have learned about personal space. The professional may want to ask questions related to everyone needing a different amount of personal space. This insight is important for group members to know in order to have appropriate physical boundaries with peers. Application of this activity can be repeated at home to ensure success.

Social Skills Group Session Four

Length

Based on a one-hour group session

About this week's group

The professional should continue to take note of any specific information they want to cover in this group session, as well as review and prep for the session. Prep would include having an alternative item (sock, for example) in case any member is uncomfortable taking off their shoe for the icebreaker. Having a general joy or sorrow ready to share and having a goodbye song ready to share. Materials for this session should be created and displayed. The icebreaker and closing activity should be practiced and the Session Overview Form ready to give to parents.

Welcome icebreaker

Each group member keeps one of their shoes on and takes the other shoe off. All of the off shoes go into a pile. If there are an odd number of members, the professional should put one shoe in the pile also. The professional then mixes up the shoes and chooses a group member to go first. The first group member closes their eyes and picks a shoe. The member then finds who the shoe belongs to and asks that person a question of their choosing. Play continues until everyone has asked a question. If a group member chooses their own shoe, the professional can decide if they should try again or share one statement about themselves.

Anything to share

The professional should follow the same suggestions from group session one or two.

Implement the social skills intervention

The professional can use the interventions provided in this session or one of their own.

Process and application of the intervention

An example of processing and application is provided at the end of each social skill intervention description.

Goodbye ritual

Teach the members a simple goodbye song they can sing. There are many online songs to choose from, or members can create their own.

Give form to parents

As the children leave the group session, the professional should give each parent the Session Overview Form. The professional will want to have the form completed prior to the group.

GROUP SESSION FOUR EXAMPLE SOCIAL SKILLS INTERVENTION FOR CHILDREN

Activity: Symphony Composers

Social Skills Target Area(s)

Including others, following rules, cooperating and participating with peers

Level

Children

Materials Needed

A bell set (one bell needed for each group member), color stickers if bells are not a variety of colors (one color for each participant), construction paper (one color that corresponds with each color sticker or bell)

Introduction

This is a great activity to do with individuals who are not sensitive to sound. A good idea is for the professional to first be the conductor while the children get used to the idea of the game, then later they can take turns being the conductor. The focus is not on the music created but the idea of focusing, working together, and participating in a fun activity. This activity allows for structured group participation and creativity. It allows clients to have some flexibility with instrument selection but provides a safe control in a social setting. Clients are able to practice focus, eye contact, group participation, following rules, and other valuable social skills.

Instructions

1. The professional should have bells displayed on a table. Each group member should pick one bell.
2. Once the bells are chosen, the professional puts a different color sticker onto each bell. There should be only one color of sticker on each bell that is being used. (This step is not needed if different color bells are being used.)
3. The professional lays out each corresponding piece of matching color construction paper in front of them. The professional then explains that whichever piece of paper they hold up, that corresponding bell should be played. The group may need to decide how each bell will be played (one gong, several rings, etc.)

4. The professional holds up a piece of paper and waits for the corresponding bell to play. The professional continues holding up various colors of paper until all group members have had a turn and have been successful with playing at the appropriate time.
5. Individual group members can take turns being the conductor while the professional can choose a bell to play.

Processing and Application

Processing questions can include what they enjoyed and did not enjoy about this activity. Discussion may be needed about noise volume and any sensitivities group members may have had. This could be replicated at home, either with various instruments, or home-made instruments (spoons, coffee cans, dried beans put in a jar, etc.)

GROUP SESSION FOUR EXAMPLE SOCIAL SKILLS INTERVENTION FOR ADOLESCENTS

For this group day, *Symphony Composers* is a great activity for adolescents as well. The professional can modify this activity by adding a variety of instruments instead of just the bells. The professional can also allow more time for the adolescent group members to be the composers, and the group members can also video one of their songs.

Social Skills Group Session Five

Length

Based on a one-hour group session

About this week's group

The professional should continue to take note of any specific information they want to cover in this group session, as well as review and prep for the session. Prep would include having animal cards or creating them with index cards. Having a general joy or sorrow ready to share or possibly have a picture of the yoga "prayer pose" to help with goodbye the ritual. Materials for this session should be created and displayed. The icebreaker and closing activity should be practiced and the Session Overview Form ready to give to parents.

Welcome icebreaker

By group session five members most likely will feel more comfortable with each other. This is a great time to introduce a fun activity like *Animal Charades*. It can be adapted for younger children by having them pick a card with an animal on it, then the group member makes noises like that animal for others to guess. With older children and adolescents, players will act out silently whatever animal card they choose.

Anything to share

The professional should follow the same suggestions from group session one or two.

Implement the social skills intervention

The professional can use the interventions provided for this session or one of their own.

Process and application of the intervention

An example of processing and application is provided at the end of each social skill intervention description.

Goodbye ritual

Before they leave, group members form a circle, put their hands together (prayer pose) and give each other a bow. Group members then put their hands up to their sides, palms facing out, connect palms with other group members, and bow.

Give form to parents

As the children leave the group session, the professional should give each parent the Session Overview Form. The professional will want to have the form completed prior to the group.

GROUP SESSION FIVE EXAMPLE SOCIAL SKILLS INTERVENTION FOR CHILDREN

Activity: Monster Maker

Social Skills Target Area(s)

Socializing with peers, including others, and following rules

Level

Children

Materials Needed

Two foam dice (the professional ahead of time writes the numbers one through six on one die; the words or pictures "eye," "ear," "nose," "mouth," "hands," and "feet" on the other die). One piece of paper with an oval, circle, square, etc. to represent the monster's body, one pencil for each group member.

Introduction

This is a fun activity that presents a small amount of challenge due to working with a non-realistic monster. Clients who may feel unskilled at drawing may seem more eager to attempt it when it is simple body parts to be drawn. Participants need to work on accepting the number that is rolled, taking turns on the rolling, and discussing the strengths and challenges with more or less sensory body parts than the monster has compared to them.

Instructions

1. The professional explains that each group member will take turns rolling both dice. Once rolled, a number and body part will be shown.
2. Whatever number is rolled, the group member draws that many body parts onto the monster template.
3. Play continues until all body parts have been represented. Group members get to decide if one particular body part is rolled more than once if they roll again or keep adding that body part to the monster.
4. Group members can choose to color the monster when completed.
5. The professional leads a discussion on the strengths and challenges this monster would have with the number of each body part.

Processing and Application

Processing questions may include asking how group members felt about having to work together on this activity. Were there any new discoveries made about working in a group? What was easier to accomplish and what was more difficult? This activity can be repeated at home with a variety of different fantasy animals and characters.

**GROUP SESSION FIVE EXAMPLE SOCIAL SKILLS
INTERVENTION FOR ADOLESCENTS**

Activity: Monster Collaborative Drawing

Social Skills Target Area(s)

Socializing with peers, including others, and following rules

Level

Adolescents

Materials Needed

One piece of paper for each group member, one pencil, a timer (may not
be needed)

Introduction

This is a great activity for group members to learn to work with others
and compromise on ideas. It also allows them to see how being flexible
and part of a team can create something really fun and special.

Instructions

1. The professional will give one piece of paper and a pencil to each
   group member. The group members should be sitting in a circle.
2. The professional will ask each group member to fold their papers
   into half (top to bottom) and then into half again (top to bottom).
   The paper should then be opened (paper should now be in four sec-
   tions, from top to bottom).
3. The professional will tell each group member to draw a monster
   head, however they like, in the very top section. They will want to
   also draw a neck that ends a bit over the second section of the paper
   (right past the first crease). The professional can choose to set a timer
   for this or not.
4. The professional will then have each group member fold the first
   section of the paper in the opposite direction so that the head is now
   hidden (but a portion of the neck can still be seen).
5. The group members will then pass their papers on to the person on
   their left. This time the professional will have each person draw a
   torso of a monster (chest, arms, hands, and stomach) on the second
   section of the paper. The professional will instruct the group members

to have the bottom of the stomach go slightly over the crease into the third section of the paper.

6. Repeat the process of folding in the opposite direction, passing to the group member on the left, and repeating, with the third section being a monster's legs, and the fourth section being a monster's feet.

7. Once the drawings are complete, open each one to see what silly monsters have been created!

Processing and Application

Discuss with the group members what they enjoyed about this activity and what they had difficulty with. Encourage them to share ways they may have struggled working in a group. Process with the group members the times and places where they will need the social skill of working in a group. This activity could be repeated at home with other types of fantasy animals and characters.

Social Skills Group Session Six

Length

Based on a one-hour group session

About this week's group

The professional should continue to take note of any specific information they want to cover in this group session, as well as review and prep for the session. Prep would include possibly having adjective examples to help with the icebreaker activity and having a general joy or sorrow ready to share. Materials for this session should be created and displayed. The icebreaker and closing activity should be practiced and the Session Overview Form ready to give to parents.

Welcome icebreaker

Nifty Names icebreaker has each group member say their name and what letter it begins with. The other group members come up with positive adjectives that begin with each group members' name. Each group member chooses the adjective they like the best and writes it on a name tag for them to wear.

Anything to share

The professional should follow the same suggestions from group session one or two.

Implement the social skills intervention

The professional can use the intervention provided for session six or one of their own.

Process and application of the intervention

An example of processing and application is provided at the end of each social skill intervention description.

Goodbye ritual

Each group member takes a turn saying goodbye to the other group members by using each of their new, nifty names.

Give form to parents

As the children leave the group session, the professional should give each parent the Session Overview Form. The professional will want to have the form completed prior to the group.

GROUP SESSION SIX EXAMPLE SOCIAL SKILLS INTERVENTION FOR CHILDREN

Activity: Topic Tower Builders (children's version)

Social Skills Target Area(s)

Having a conversation, sharing with others, listening without interrupting, expressing opinions, and participating in a group

Level

Children

Materials

Colored blocks (around eight to ten blocks per group member)

Introduction

Children with autism often love to share information but may monopolize the conversation on a given topic. This game allows each group member to share facts and opinions about animals in a fair way. It will also encourage active listening when not speaking.

Instructions

1. The professional puts out the tub of colored blocks and has each group member choose eight to ten. The professional tells the group that they can pick whatever colors they want.
2. All group members will sit in a circle with a sturdy surface in the middle (a surface that will allow blocks to stand on top of each other). The professional explains that they are going to call out an animal and a color. The color called out will be one of the block colors.
3. The first group member, if they have that color, will place the block down, then say one thing related to that animal. If they do not have that color, they will skip to the next person. If they have more than one block of that color, they only put one block down and waits for their next turn.
4. Each group member continues in this matter, stacking their block onto the previous one, until all of the color blocks are used.
5. The game is continued, with the professional calling out an animal and a color, until all blocks are used or the tower falls. If the tower falls, group members can decide if they would like to count the blocks and improve their score.

Processing and Application

Discussion can include what are facts vs. opinions, similarities and differences between group members' statements, and how they handled waiting their turn, or the tower falling. Group members can discuss where it may be important to be able to display these social skills.

GROUP SESSION SIX EXAMPLE SOCIAL SKILLS INTERVENTION FOR ADOLESCENTS

Activity: Topic Tower Builders (adolescent version)

Social Skill Target Area(s)

Having a conversation, sharing with others, listening without interrupting, expressing opinions, and participating in a group

Level

Adolescents

Materials Needed

Colored blocks and index cards with a subject of group interest made by the professional

Introduction

This is a great activity to allow group members to share their facts and opinions on various topics, without monopolizing the conversation. It is structured in a way that one idea is shared at a time, while a block is added to the tower. Many individuals with autism enjoy sharing facts on preferred topics but may struggle discussing non-preferred ones. It can also be difficult for them to determine when to allow for their peers to comment. This activity is structured in a way that allows clients to practice discussing preferred topics one statement at a time, while listening as well to what others think. It also introduces the idea of discussing non-preferred topics, an essential social skill.

Instructions

1. The professional creates a deck of cards, each with a topic on it. The professional needs to make sure the topics chosen are of interest to the clients and well-known to them.
2. The professional sets out blocks and subject cards. He or she explains that the youngest person starts first, by choosing a subject card. Once a card is chosen, the player chooses a block, sets the block on the table or floor, and states one fact or opinion about the subject.
3. Play continues in a clockwise order with each player choosing a block, setting it on top of the tower while sharing one fact or opinion about the subject.

4. Each player is allowed one "pass" if he or she cannot come up with a fact or opinion.
5. Each player can only share one fact or opinion at a time; no one can go twice in a row.
6. The tower is built when all passes have been used and there is no way to continue sharing without a player going twice. Blocks are counted to see how big of a conversation tower was built. If the tower falls, group members can decide if they would like to count the blocks and improve their score.

Processing and Application

Processing involves any possible difficulty with taking turns. The professional may also want to ask if there was any frustration if the tower fell. The professional may wish to review what facts and opinions are and spend some time discussing why it is important to know the difference between the two. Parents could practice fact versus opinion at home both in natural conversation and in game play.

Social Skills Group Session Seven

Length

Based on a one-hour group session

About this week's group

The professional should continue to take note of any specific information they want to cover in this group session, as well as review and prep for the session. Prep would include having index cards ready with each group member's name for the icebreaker and having a general joy or sorrow ready to share. Materials for this session should be created and displayed. The icebreaker and closing activity should be practiced and the Session Overview Form ready to give to parents.

Welcome icebreaker

Name Game icebreaker involves having each group member's name on an index card. Group members pick one index card, then walk around the room finding three to five things that share the first initial with the card they chose (example: if "Sam" is the card chosen, the child may pick up a "scarf"). Once everyone has picked items, group members have to guess which name each person had.

Anything to share

The professional should follow the same suggestions from group session one or two.

Implement the social skills intervention

The professional can use the interventions provided for this session or one of their own.

Process and application of the intervention

An example of processing and application is provided at the end of each social skill intervention description.

Goodbye ritual

Group members take turns hooking their pinky fingers with another group members and giving a goodbye shake.

Give form to parents

As the children leave the group session, the professional should give each parent the Session Overview Form. The professional will want to have the form completed prior to the group.

GROUP SESSION SEVEN EXAMPLE SOCIAL SKILLS INTERVENTION FOR CHILDREN

Activity: Where It Belongs (children version)

Social Skills Target Area(s)

Knowing safety information, knowing appropriate hygiene, knowing home and school norms, and compromising

Level

Children

Materials

Four pieces of construction paper hung up in each corner of the room. One piece says "home," one piece says "school," one piece says "store," one piece says "outside" (for younger children, pictures instead of the words may be more helpful).

Introduction

This activity involves movement which can be regulating for children. The children will be thinking on their feet while moving, which can be essential in other areas of their lives. They may also encounter having to decide on one place to stand when more than one option makes sense to them. This discernment can be difficult for children with autism but practicing during game play is helpful.

Instructions

1. The professional explains that they are going to call out something that children do. When they do, the group members should walk to the corner of the room with the sign that says the place where it would be appropriate to do this. The professional explains that there may be more than one acceptable place, but the children must choose one.
2. The professional then calls out up to 20 things that children do (examples include eating dessert, yelling, dancing, paying attention, taking off clothes, etc.) and gives group members time to walk to their corner.
3. The group members explain why they chose to stand where they did.

Processing and Application

Children can process with the professional why they chose to stand where they did and hear why others chose their particular places to stand. Discussion can include any difficulties in choosing between more than one acceptable place in the game. This game can easily be practiced at home as well.

GROUP SESSION SEVEN EXAMPLE SOCIAL SKILLS INTERVENTION FOR ADOLESCENTS

Activity: Where it Belongs (adolescent version)

Social Skill Target Area

Knowing safety information, knowing appropriate hygiene, knowing home and school norms, and compromising

Level

Adolescents

Materials

Magazine pictures of places taped around the therapy room (good suggestions are bathroom, kitchen, classroom, bedroom, playground, store, doctor's office, etc.), 20 slips of paper with verbs written on them hidden around the playroom (good suggestions are "yelling," "laughing," "whispering," "taking off clothes," "running," etc.), and tape

Introduction

Problem solving is an essential skill for adolescents, and adolescents with autism may find this difficult to do in a group. Practicing working in a group is a great way to help these adolescents feel more comfortable and confident with their decision-making skills.

Instructions

1. The professional explains that there are 20 slips of paper around the room. Group members can work individually, in partners, or in teams to find all 20 slips of paper.
2. Once all 20 are found group members work individually, in partners, or as one team to read the verb on the slip of paper, then choose which place taped on the wall would be the best place to do this verb. If working with another person, they need to decide on one place together. They then tape the slip of paper onto the place and tell the group why they made their choice.
3. When completed, the professional makes copies of each page (with the slips of paper still on them) for each client to have their own book to take home to review.

Processing and Application

This activity allows for discussion on social skills in a fun, game-like way. The group members may feel like they are understood and not alone in any difficulties they may have when learning from the other adolescents. The extra take home makes for further practice on where certain activities should be done and the appropriateness or inappropriateness of certain behaviors in certain environments.

Social Skills Group Session Eight

Length

Based on a one-hour group session

About this week's group

The professional should continue to take note of any specific information they want to cover in this group session, as well as review and prep for the session. Prep would include practicing singing the song for the icebreaker and have a general joy or sorrow ready to share. Materials for this session should be created and displayed. The icebreaker and closing activity should be practiced and the Session Overview Form ready to give to parents.

Welcome icebreaker

The professional explains that every time they say a word beginning with the letter *B*, the group members are to stand if seated, and sit down if standing. Then the professional sings, "Bring Back My Bonny."

> "My Bonny lies over the ocean. My Bonny lies over the sea.
> My Bonny lies over the ocean. Oh, bring back my Bonny to me.
> Bring back, bring back, bring back my Bonny to me, to me.
> Bring back, bring back, oh, bring back my Bonny to me."

Anything to share

The professional should follow the same suggestions from group session one or two.

Implement the social skills intervention

The professional can use the interventions provided for session eight or one of their own.

Process and application of the intervention

An example of processing and application is provided at the end of each social skill intervention description.

Goodbye ritual

The professional can repeat the game *Bring Back My Bonny*, which helps the group members improve in their ability to listen and is a fun way to end the session.

Give form to parents

As the children leave the group session, the professional should give each parent the Session Overview Form. The professional will want to have the form completed prior to the group.

GROUP SESSION EIGHT EXAMPLE SOCIAL SKILLS INTERVENTION FOR CHILDREN

Activity: Move It! Move It!

Social Skill Target Area

Socializing with others, following rules of a group, and participating with peers

Level

Children

Materials

Foam die (the professional writes the word or picture "head," "shoulders," "arms," "hands," "legs," "feet" on each side of the dice), and a music source.

Introduction

Movement is an important part of regulation. This intervention is best saved for the ending group sessions since there is a degree of vulnerably with dancing. Group members by now will most likely be much more comfortable with each other. Getting in touch with their body, learning where their body is in relation to space, and actually moving their bodies in a variety of ways can be very helpful to clients. The idea of clients dancing in front of a group may feel intimidating but breaking down movement in this way can feel safer and more fun.

Instructions

1. The professional chooses music to listen to that the group members enjoy.
2. The professional rolls the die. Whichever body part is shown, that is the only body part the members move.
3. Members continue to move previous body part while die continues to be rolled. If the same body part is rolled again, group members get to change up how they are moving that body part.
4. The dance is created once all body parts are moving.

Processing and Application

The professional can process with the group how they felt dancing in front of other group members. The children can be praised for their brave dancing. Movement can be discussed as an essential way to regulate when feeling worried or stressed. Invite the group members to practice some of these moves when they are feeling dysregulated in other environments.

GROUP SESSION EIGHT EXAMPLE SOCIAL SKILLS INTERVENTION FOR ADOLESCENTS

Activity: Group High Five

Social Skill Target Area

Socializing with others, following rules of a group, and participating with peers

Level

Adolescents

Materials

None

Introduction

This is a whole group activity where the members form and sit in a circle. It typically works best if group members are sitting on a floor. The professional should join the circle and participate in the activity. *Group High Five* can last as long as the members want to play and can have many variations.

Instructions

1. The professional has the group participants sit in a circle (ideally on the floor).
2. The professional explains they are going to play a game where they pass a high five around the circle.
3. The professional should begin by giving a normal high five to the person sitting to their right and then that person continues the high five around the group circle until it gets back to the professional.
4. At this point, the professional explains that each member will send around a high five but should make a variation on the move, maybe a double high five, a pinky high five, up high/down low, with your thumbs, standing up, etc. Whatever the participant can think of, the group can do.
5. The next person to go is the person sitting to the left of the professional. This person can decide what type of high five to do and start it around the circle. Once it has gotten back to him or her, the next person can go.

6. This continues until each member has had a turn creating a high five to send around the group circle.
7. One fun variation is to try and keep all the high fives going in unison. Another variation would be to add a reverse call out—anyone at any time can say "reverse" and the direction must change. The professional can be creative and think of many variations to this activity.

Processing and Application

Once the activity has been completed, the professional can process with the group how it felt to participate. Some processing questions might include did you feel uncomfortable connecting with other people? What felt challenging? Was there anything about the activity that felt good or fun? Have you ever had to do anything with a group and what was the experience like?

Social Skills Group Session Nine

Length

Based on a one-hour group session

About this week's group

The professional should continue to take note of any specific information they want to cover in this group session, as well as review and prep for the session. Prep would include possibly having picture examples of essential items for the icebreaker activity and having a general joy or sorrow ready to share. Materials for this session should be created and displayed. The icebreaker and closing activity should be practiced and the Session Overview Form ready to give to parents.

Welcome icebreaker

The professional has the children pretend that the group has been stranded on a deserted island. They must work together to come up with one item each person has that can help the group survive as a whole. This activity can be spent talking or drawing items on paper.

Anything to share

The professional should follow the same suggestions from group session one or two.

Implement the social skills intervention

The professional can use the interventions provided for session nine or one of their own.

Process and application of the intervention

An example of processing and application is provided at the end of each social skill intervention description.

Goodbye ritual

Since this is the second to last session, the professional may want to take the last five minutes to discuss the group coming to an end. The professional may get ideas about celebration treats they may want or special activities they may want to do in the last session.

Give form to parents

As the children leave the group session, the professional should give each parent the Session Overview Form. The professional will want to have the form completed prior to the group.

GROUP SESSION NINE EXAMPLE SOCIAL SKILLS INTERVENTION FOR CHILDREN

A ctivity: Scavenger Hunt

Social Skill Target Area

Participating in a group, compromising, safety needs, and problem solving

Level

Children

Materials

None

Introduction

This activity allows group members to problem solve both real and not so real situations. It can help with making choices and working with others to come to a decision. Having a visual object the participants are looking for helps make this activity easier to complete.

Instructions

1. The professional explains to group members that any object in the room can be used for this activity (unless certain items should be off limits, for example items on therapist's desk).
2. The professional has the group work individually, in partner groups, or as one team to choose one item in the room that would be the best used in a particular situation. Situations should be a mix of realistic and fantasy.
3. Once members have chosen the object, they explain to the professional, or other group members why the object was chosen.

Examples of situations

*   You need to give a gift to a three-year-old.
*   You need to fight a zombie.
*   You have a play date with a friend.
*   You need to fall asleep.
*   You have to walk in the rain.
*   You have to take a bath.

Processing and Application

Processing can occur during the activity to highlight the differences in opinion. Since the children have been processing verbally during this intervention, less time would be needed on processing after the activity.

GROUP SESSION NINE EXAMPLE SOCIAL SKILLS INTERVENTION FOR ADOLESCENTS

Activity: Domino Challenge

Social Skill Target Area

Following rules, working as a team, compromise, socializing with peers, and expressing ideas

Level

Adolescents

Materials

Colored Dominoes (the professional can use traditional dominoes that have different colored dots on each one, or can purchase plastic dominoes that are a variety of colors)

Introduction

Domino Challenge is an excellent way to work with structure, challenge, patience, and more. Often the dominoes fall before the track is complete, and players have to persevere and keep going. This is a great activity to also show how individual work can also be part of a greater picture.

Instructions

1. Group members are divided into teams based on however many colors of dominos are being used (example: if the professional has blue, green, yellow, and red dominos, there would be four teams.) If the professional is using standard white dominos, he or she would need to add colored sticker dots to differentiate the teams.
2. The instruction is for each team to create a track of their choice with their color of dominos. The goal is to have a starting domino, that when pressed with a finger, will create a unison of the dominos falling. The team members should work together to create a domino track of their choosing (they can choose a simple straight line or can create a more elaborate path).
3. Once each team is successful with their domino tracks (meaning each team has had their dominos all fall down), the new challenge is for the entire group to work together to have a large domino track with all of the colors combined. Group members can decide to either

stay in their teams and create connecting paths or combine all of the dominos and work as one team to create the path together.

4. Once completed, the professional can tip the first domino over to see if all the dominos fall!

Processing and Application

Processing may include any frustration felt while working with the dominoes. Group members should be praised for not giving up. Examples of other times and situations where persevering may be highlighted.

Social Skills Group Session Ten

Length

Based on a one-hour group session

About this week's group

The professional should continue to take note of any specific information they want to cover in this group session, as well as review and prep for the session. Prep would include having celebration foods ready to be shared and having a goodbye take home object for the group members. Materials for this session should be created and displayed. The icebreaker and closing activity should be practiced and the Session Overview Form ready to give to parents.

Welcome icebreaker

The professional prompts group members to think of one word to describe the 10-week group. It can be any word of their choosing (how they felt, what they learned, etc.) Each group member will share the word they chose and why they chose it.

Anything to share

The professional should follow the same suggestions from group session one or two.

Implement the social skills intervention

The professional can use the interventions provided for this session or one of their own.

Process and application of the intervention

An example of processing and application is provided at the end of each social skill intervention description.

Goodbye ritual

The therapist should have a small take home for the group members which can be given to them at this time. Examples include a goodie bag of candy, a photo frame with a picture of the group, etc.

Give form to parents

As the children leave the group session, the professional should give each parent the Session Overview Form. The professional will want to have the form completed prior to the group.

GROUP SESSION TEN EXAMPLE SOCIAL SKILLS INTERVENTION FOR CHILDREN

Activity: Fill My Bucket

Social Skills Target Area

Verbally expressing feelings, connecting with peers, following directions, and showing empathy

Level

Children

Materials

The book *Have You Filled A Bucket Today?* by Carol McCloud, one small bucket for each group member (they will get to take these home), name tag stickers, permanent market, index cards, and pencils

Introduction

This book is fantastic for every professional to have. Many schools have purchased this book for character building lessons, so children may be familiar with it. This activity allows group members to share with each other and have a take-home object to help them remember the group.

Instructions

1. The professional reads the book *Have You Filled A Bucket Today?* to the group members.
2. The group processes the book. Sample questions include:
   a. Can you give an example of how you filled someone's bucket during this group?
   b. Can you think of a time where you may have taken from someone's bucket during this group?
   c. Can you give an example of when someone filled your bucket during this group?
   d. Is there a way we can continue to fill our group members' buckets even though group is ending?
3. The professional gives each child a small bucket, a name tag sticker and a permanent market. The professional asks each group member to put their name on the sticker and attach it to their bucket.
4. The professional then instructs each child to place their buckets on a table, ledge, etc.

5. The professional hands out index cards to each group member (they will need one card for each group member, including themselves) and a pencil. The group members should write one positive thing about each group member, including themselves. It is helpful to have them first write the group member's name on the index card, so the cards don't get mixed up. The professional can help with writing if necessary.
6. The group members fill each other's buckets, placing the written index card into each group member's buckets. The professional can have the group members read during the group, or at home.

Processing and Application

Termination groups can be very difficult on children, especially those who have had difficulty making and keeping friends. The professional should have extra time allotted during the group session to further process the feelings of the group terminating.

GROUP SESSION TEN SOCIAL SKILLS INTERVENTION FOR ADOLESCENTS

Activity: Secret Message

Social Skill Target Area(s)

Talking about feelings, sharing with others, and showing empathy

Level

Adolescents

Materials

Lemon juice, cotton swabs, white construction paper cut into fourths, markers, and hair dryer

Introduction

This activity is great for adolescents since they often get embarrassed complimenting others or being complimented. The invisible ink gives them a level of privacy that can be important for them. This is also science based, which many adolescents with autism enjoy.

Instructions

1. The professional begins by stating this is their final group session. He or she allows the adolescents to process their feelings about this. Questions may include:
    a. What is one positive thing you experienced about group?
    b. Is there an "oops" you may have committed during group you would like to acknowledge and apologize for?
    c. What was the most fun activity?
    d. How do you feel you have improved socially?
    e. Is there a way you all can stay connected even though group is over?

2. The professional instructs the group to think about each group member, and positive things about them. These can be discussed out loud or processed internally.

3. The professional gives each group member a small bowl of lemon juice, a marker, a few cotton swabs, and several pieces of white construction paper already cut into four smaller pieces. The group

members will write one group member's name on each piece of paper (including themselves).

4. Group members will now write one word describing each group member using the invisible ink! They simply have to dip their cotton swab into the lemon juice, then write the word on the paper.
5. When finished each group member is given the papers with their names on it. Group members take turns using the hair dryer to discover each of their positive traits.

Processing and Application

Termination groups can be very difficult on adolescents, especially those who have had difficulty making and keeping friends. The professional should have extra time allotted during the group session to further process the feelings of the group terminating.

7 Additional Social Skills Interventions for Children and Adolescents

SOCIAL SKILLS INTERVENTIONS FOR CHILDREN

Activity: Find the Prize

Social Skill Target Area(s)

Listening, following instructions, and turn taking

Level

Children

Materials

Several small prizes (candy, small toys, stickers, etc.)

Introduction

This activity helps children learn listening skills and helps them follow verbal directions. The child has to listen to the professional's instruction in order to find their prize. Children participate one at a time which allows for practicing waiting and turn taking. The professional may have to remind children to wait and listen and keep children focused on the goals they are working on in this activity.

Instructions

1. Before the group meets, the professional hides some small prizes around the group room (usually pieces of candy, stickers, or small toys, enough so there is one for each child in the group). The prizes should be hidden so they are not easy to find.
2. The professional tells the groups they are going to play a game where they try to find some prizes that are hidden around the group room.

3. The professional explains that each child will take a turn and search for a prize in the room. Once a child has found a prize, their turn is over, and the next child gets to search.
4. The child must listen to the professional as the professional gives the child directions to help them discover where the prize is hidden. The professional should give simple directions, one direction at a time that progressively leads the child to the prize. For example, a prize may be hidden in a sand tray. The professional might say, "Look for something that is rectangle shaped." "Now look for something that you can find at a beach." "Now put your hands in the thing you might find at the beach and feel around."
5. The professional keeps producing simple directions until the child finds the prize. At this point that child's turn is over and another child goes next. This keeps happening until each child in the group finds a prize.
6. While a child is taking their tun, the other children are watching and listing.

Processing and Application

This activity presents a fun and exciting process for working on important social skills such as turn taking, waiting patiently, and listening to instructions. Once each child has completed their turn, the professional should ask the group what the most challenging part of the activity was and what was the easiest part. The professional should also share their observations of what children seemed to struggle with and what seemed easy. The professional should ask the participants what places in their lives they must wait, take turns, and listen and encourage the participants to focus on being successful in those places just as they were with this activity.

Activity: Space Mistakes

Social Skill Target Area(s)

Understanding personal space and boundaries

Level

Children

Materials

White paper, crayons or markers

Introduction

This activity helps children understand and practice personal boundaries and personal space issues. Children have the opportunity to practice with each other and the professional. The professional should begin with a brief and simple explanation of what personal space and boundaries mean. The professional should complete a list of personal space and boundary situations to practice. These should be target issues the participants struggle with; some examples might include standing too close to others, touching others, appropriate voice volume, waiting in lines, touching other people's things, and wondering away from groups or adults.

Instructions

1. Prior to the group meeting, the professional creates a list of personal space mistakes and public boundary mistakes.
2. The professional reads and describes the list to the children.
3. The children have to show the professional an example of the mistakes, and then show the professional the correct thing to do instead. The children will do this through role play.
4. Each child in the group takes a turn and chooses something from the list. The professional can participate with the child in the role play and the professional will likely have to demonstrate appropriate responses through the role play. Some participants may not know what an appropriate response would be.
5. Once everything on the list is completed, participants can receive a small reward such as a sticker or piece of candy.

Processing and Application

Once the items on the list have all be role played, the professional should ask the participants to share if they have struggled with any of these areas. The professional can also ask the participants to talk about what they think is the hardest thing to do and what seems easy. The professional can talk about the importance of understanding boundaries and personal space when interacting with others and in public situations. The professional can encourage the participants to think about times and places they may be the next day when they could practice the appropriate responses that were covered in the group meeting.

Activity: Roles and Turns

Social Skill Target Area(s)

Turn taking, being a part of a group, playing with and supporting others

Level

Children

Materials

Several balls that can be tossed or kicked back and forth (preferably soft/cloth balls)

Introduction

This activity addresses several social skill areas. The participants complete the activity as a group with each person having a role in the group. Through the activity they practice working together as a group, taking turns, and encouraging each other. The professional may participate and role model but will certainly want to observe and make sure the participants are being effective in their group roles. This activity can be repeated several times and can be adapted to multiple variations of the same basic concept. It typically requires some space for children to move around but one variation for limited space might be having the children sit at a table and roll a marble to each other.

Instructions

1. The professional explains to the group they are going to be playing a game using some balls they will be throwing back and forth.
2. The professional should have a couple of balls (not enough for everyone).
3. Ideally the children are put in groups of three. If needed, the professional can participate in a group. The professional should adjust this activity for the number of participants in the group.
4. Two of the participants in the group of three are chosen to start first by throwing the ball back and forth to each other while the third person in the group cheers for them.
5. They will do this for a couple of minutes, then the professional will say "switch" and the participants will rotate their position, so the person who was cheering now throws the ball back and forth with one of the other participants and a new person cheers for them.

6. After about two minutes, the professional says "switch" and the participants rotate their position again. This happens until each participant has been in the cheering position. If applicable, the activity can be repeated.

Processing and Application

The time of throwing the ball (which could also be kicking a ball back and forth or any variation) should be keep short to keep the children interested and avoid a meltdown. The child in the cheering position could also be given the task of keeping track of the time. This activity can be done with other things besides balls (balloons, bubble blowing, etc.). Once the activity has been completed, the professional should ask the group participants what it felt like to participate as a group and have specific group roles. The professional can also ask the participants to share about a time they had to do something with a group and share about what they have learned that could help them the next time they have to participate with a group of peers.

Activity: Animal Pairs

Social Skill Target Area(s)

Introducing self and paying attention to others

Level

Children

Materials

Index cards and markers

Introduction

This activity focuses on helping participants pay attention to others, notice others, and the beginnings of engaging with another person and introducing yourself to someone else. These skills are addressed in a fun and interactive manner using a matching game concept. The instructions use animals for the index card matching game, but anything could be chosen—toys, sports, food, video game titles, etc. If there is something that might be more engaging for the group, then the professional should choose that for the matching portion. Professionals should keep the process fun and simple as some children may feel uncomfortable with the group social interaction.

Instructions

1. Prior to the group meeting, the professional will make index cards with animal names written on them or pictures of animals on them (pictures for younger children or if there are children in the group who cannot read). The professional makes two matching sets for each animal.
2. The professional explains to the group they are going to play a matching game where each participant will have to find their matching animal pair.
3. The professional passes out the index cards to the children. Make sure that everyone has a match and make sure the children do not reveal what they are.
4. The professional will explain to the children that there is another child with the same animal, and they are going to find out who is their match by acting like the animal on their card and observing what the other children are acting like.

5. When the professional says "go" the children have to act like the animal on their card and/or make the sound of the animal on their card and find the other child who has their matching animal.
6. Once all the matches have been discovered, the activity can be played a second time with new animal index cards passed out to the participants.
7. If needed, the professional can also participate and have an animal card and try to find their match.

Processing and Application

This activity involves the whole group and has some animated and interactive elements that may be challenging for some of the group participants. The professional should be very observant of each of the participants and how they are handling the activity. Once the game has been completed, the professional should ask the group how it felt to participate in this activity—what felt comfortable and what felt uncomfortable? The professional can also ask the group to share about any times they remember interacting with others and it felt uncomfortable.

Activity: Bingo Friends

Social Skill Target Area(s)

Making friends, asking questions, and getting to know others

Level

Children

Materials

Bingo card template and markers (Table 7.1 provides a sample bingo card)

Introduction

This activity works on noticing others, asking questions, remembering others, and making friends. This activity requires the participants to interact at a fairly high level and ask each other questions. This may be uncomfortable for some participants and the professional will want to be observant of each participant's process and assist any child who may need help. This is a fun group activity which helps children understand processes involved in meeting and getting to know other children. The activity can be repeated in additional group meetings with the professional creating new bingo cards.

Instructions

1. The professional will create simple bingo cards on pieces of paper before the group begins. On the bingo cards should be various identifying information about all the children in the group such as has brown hair, is eight years old, likes Minecraft, etc. The card can have more squares than the number of members in the group, but each item written in a square should be something that there will be a match for with at least one of the group members.
2. The professional will share with the group that they will be playing a bingo game.
3. The professional explains that they will pass out a bingo card to each participant and the cards will have squares on them with something written in each square.
4. When the professional says "go" the participants must interact with each other and try to find someone who matches what is written on one of the bingo card squares. One child could be a match for more than one square.

5. When they find someone who matches one or more of the statements on the bingo card, they should try to remember who it is by writing down their name on the card or some other identifying information.
6. The game continues until each participant has found a match for each square on their Bingo card.
7. Once everyone has finished, each participant can share their card, indicating who in the group they found for each matching statement on the card.
8. The professional can also participate in this activity and there can be something written in one of the squares on the bingo card that is about the professional.

Processing and Application

This activity involves a great deal of social skill work. If the professional is comfortable, he or she could provide the participants with a small prize once the activity has been completed. The professional should ask the participants how they felt about completing this activity—what felt uncomfortable, what part was difficult, what felt comfortable, did something feel fun? The professional can also ask the participants to share about struggles they have had with meeting other children or trying to participate with other children in a group activity. The professional should also encourage the participants to think about how they could continue to practice ways to feel more comfortable meeting new people and interacting with peers in a group setting.

Table 7.1 Bingo Card Example

Is 10 years old	Has brown hair	Likes video games
Has blue eyes	Has a brother	Hates math
Likes pizza	Plays Minecraft	Has a pet dog

Activity: Bubbles Social Skills (Grant, 2017)

Social Skill Target Area(s)

Asking questions, sharing, turn taking, and general manners

Level

Children

Materials

Bubbles, one bottle for every two participants

Introduction

This activity uses bubbles to engage participants in practicing various social skills that may need improvement. The professional can create several different social scripts or situations using a bubble blowing process to practice the social skills. The professional should create the social skill scripts prior to the group meeting. The scripts should address social skills that the group members need to practice.

Instructions

1. The professional explains to the participants they are going to work on increasing social skills while blowing bubbles.
2. The professional begins by reading and demonstrating a script to use with the bubbles. The professional tells the group they are going to practice implementing the script using bubble blowing.
3. The professional divides the group up into pairs and gives each pair a bottle of bubbles.
4. The professional tells the pairs to begin by blowing the bubbles and following the social skills script. They should continue going through the script and practicing until the professional tells them to stop (example scripts are provided at the end of this activity description).
5. The professional should monitor each pair and assist them if they are struggling with the script.
6. The professional should let the children practice for several minutes and when it seems like they are accomplishing the script fairly well, the professional can introduce a new social script to practice.

Processing and Application

This activity helps develop various social skills. The professional will likely need to conceptualize several different scripts and teach the scripts to the children, making sure the scripts are scenarios the child needs to work on. Once the activity has been completed, the professional should ask the group how they felt about the activity—was there any part that was challenging, any part that seemed easy? The professional can also ask the group participants if they can think of any additional social scripts the group could practice using the bubbles.

Example Social Skill Scripts

Introducing self, taking turns, and sharing: The participants take turns blowing bubbles, one turn blowing the bubbles for each person. One person starts by blowing the bubbles, the other person then says, "Hi my name is _____, can I play with the bubbles?" The bubble blower says, "Yes, I will share with you," and hands the other person the bubbles. The person receiving the bubbles says, "Thank you," and the other person says, "You are welcome." The script is then repeated with the new bubble blower and they go back and forth several times.

 Telling others you don't like something and hearing them tell you they don't like something: One person blows the bubbles; the other person says, "I don't like bubbles. Please don't blow them by me." The bubble blower says, "Sorry, I will blow them over here." Then the other person says, "Thank you." They switch roles and practice this script back and forth several times.

Activity: An Emotional Story (Grant 2017)

Social Skill Target Area(s)

Listing, considering others, and identifying emotions

Level

Children

Materials

None

Introduction

This activity helps children work on focusing and listening for key words or phrases especially related to emotions. It also helps children recognize when someone is experiencing an emotion and why another person might be experiencing a certain emotion. The professional creates one or more short stories that the professional will read to the group. The stories should have multiple examples of emotions being felt.

Instructions

1. Before the group meeting, the professional will write one to three short stories that reference people feeling various emotions (some examples are provided at the end of this activity description).
2. The professional explains to the group that they will be reading a short story and they are going to try and focus their attention on the story.
3. The professional explains that while they are reading the story, the group needs to listen, stop the professional, and identify every time an emotion is expressed in the story.
4. The participants must state what emotion is expressed, who in the story is expressing the emotion, why the person in the story is expressing the emotion, and if he or she would feel that way in the same situation.
5. These are questions that can be asked by the practitioner each time a child stops the story to identify an emotion.
6. After the story is finished, the professional can read another story or ask the participants if they want to write their own emotional story. If the participants write their own emotional story, they can then read the story and have the other group members identify the emotions.

7. When reading the story to the group, it is likely the participants will miss some emotions. The professional should stop the story and mention to the participants that there was an emotion they missed and re-read that section of the story to provide the group an opportunity to identify the missed emotion.

Processing and Application

This activity works on sharing emotional experiences as well as several other emotional regulation categories. The difficulty and length of the story should vary depending on the group members ages and functioning level. Several different stories can be written referencing many different situations and can also include social situations and challenges. Children who struggle recognizing the emotions in the story may need to start by reading the story themselves, circling all the emotions they find in the story, then discussing the emotions. Once the activity has been completed, the professional should ask the group to share how they felt about the activity—was it easy to notice the feeling, was it challenging to stay focused and listen? The professional can also ask the group members to share what they think is the most challenging thing they do where they have to stay focused and listen.

Example Emotional Story 1—Sam's First Day of School

Sam was awakened by his alarm clock. It was 7:00am and time to get up and get ready for the first day of school. Sam was feeling tired and really didn't want to get out of bed. Sam's mother told him he had to get out of bed and get dressed; she was worried he would miss the school bus. Sam got out of bed and started getting dressed. Sam was excited to see some friends he had not seen all summer but anxious that there might be a bully at school. Sam got dressed and ate his breakfast which gave him a sick feeling in his stomach. Sam continued to feel anxious as he got on the school bus. There was a lot of noise on the bus, and Sam was getting irritated by all the loudness. The bus finally got to school and Sam went into his classroom. Sam was feeling relieved to finally be at school. Sally, one of Sam's best friends, came and sat beside him. This made Sam happy, and he thought maybe school was not so bad. Sam actually started to feel excited about going to school this year even if it meant he had to get up at 7:00am every morning.

Example Emotional Story 2—Sally's Brother

Sally walked into her room ready to play with all her toys and have a lot of fun! As she walked into her room, her mood changed from excited to angry. Sally's little brother Michael was in her room, and he had broken several of her toys. Sally was so angry that she yelled at the top of her lungs for Michael to get out of her room. Michael seemed surprised and scared at the same time. Michael quickly ran out of Sally's room. As Sally looked around her room she felt sad; many of her favorite toys were broken. Sally's mother heard Sally yell at Michael and came into Sally's room. She saw Sally looking sad and upset and realized what had happened. Sally's mother told Sally that everything would be okay; they would replace all the toys that had been broken. Sally started to feel happy. Sally's mother also told Sally that they would get a special lock for her door so her brother could not get in. Sally was excited to get some new toys and relieved that her brother would not be able to get in her room.

Activity: Together Balloons

Social Skill Target Area(s)

Teamwork, communication, and playing with others

Level

Children

Materials

Balloons (one for every two group members)

Introduction

Together Balloons provides a simple, fun, and engaging way for group members to work on connecting with each other, working together to accomplish a task, and having fun together. The professional will want to make sure that no group members have an allergy to balloons or have a fear of balloons. This should be discovered prior to the group meeting and, if there is a member with one of these issues, then this activity should not be implemented.

Instructions

1. The professional explains to the group members that they will be playing a game together that involves a balloon.
2. The professional explains that they will be dividing up into pairs and each pair will have a balloon. The professional can choose the pairs and should place the children with their partner at this time.
3. The professional blows up the balloons (or may already have them prepared) and tells the children that they are going to work together with their partner to keep the balloon in the air and not hitting the ground. They are working as a team and they should help each other.
4. The children stand facing each other and grab both of each other's hands. The professional explains that they have to keep holding each other's hands the whole time that they are trying to keep the balloon in the air.
5. If the balloon hits the ground, it should be picked up and the game starts again. The activity should be played for several minutes, then the children can switch pairs and play again.
6. The professional should make sure that the children understand the activity is about having fun and not mastering keeping the balloon in the air. It is likely the balloons will hit the ground often.

Processing and Application

This activity helps children work on connection and relationship development through physical touch, working cooperatively, and attuning to and being aware of others. The professional should decide how long to play the activity and how often to switch pairs. Once the activity has ended, the professional should process with the members and ask them how they felt about the activity—was there any part of interacting with another person that was challenging, was anything easy? The professional can also ask the group participants to share about a time when they had to work with another person and what that experience was like.

Activity: Boatman

Social Skill Target Area(s)
Listening, working together, and playing with others

Level
Children

Materials
None

Introduction

This activity helps children practice playing an organized game with a group of peers. The children also work on listening and cooperation skills. The professional may participate in this game and will want to clearly go over the game rules to make sure everyone understands what they are doing. This can be a very fun and exciting game with a great deal of social interaction; thus, the professional will want to carefully monitor the participants to make sure they are managing the activity well.

Instructions

1. The professional explains that they are going to play a popular children's game called Boatman.
2. One child is chosen to be the boatman (catcher). The boatman stands in the middle of the room. The rest of the group participants choose to stand on one side or the other of the boatman. If no one wants to be the boatman, the professional can start by being the boatman.
3. When the professional says "go" the group members say together "Boatman, boatman may we cross the river?" The boatman then answers, "Only if you are . . ." and then describes a category such as ". . . wearing blue".
4. The boatman's choice of category can be as general or specific as he or she wishes.
5. All the members who meet that category have to run and cross the river to the other side without being caught. The boatman tries to touch them as they are trying to get past the boatman.
6. Any children who are caught join the boatman in the middle and help with the catching.
7. The process repeats until all the members have been caught, then a new group member can be the boatman and the game can be played again.

Processing and Application

If there is time in the group meeting, each group participate can take a turn as the boatman. If a child does not want to be the boatman, they should not be forced into that position. Once the activity has been completed, the professional should ask the members to share how they felt about playing with others in an organized game. The professional can also ask if they have every had this type of experience before and what was it like—did it go well? Was it challenging?

Activity: Safe and Unsafe

Social Skill Target Area(s)

Safety skills, listening, and paying attention

Level

Children

Materials

Paper or cardboard for each group member, and markers or pens

Introduction

This activity focuses on helping children learn about safe and unsafe situations and behaviors. The professional is encouraged to make the activity as fun and engaging as possible. It is most helpful if the professional knows about some behaviors that group members have been doing that are unsafe and targets these behaviors in the scenarios.

Instructions

1. The professional explains to the group that they are going to do an activity that focuses on learning about safe and unsafe things and behaviors.
2. The professional gives each child two pieces of paper or two pieces of cardboard. The pieces should be square pieces approximately 4″ x 4″.
3. The participants are instructed to write an S on one piece and a U on the other piece, and the children can decorate the two pieces however they want. The S stands for safe and the U stands for unsafe.
4. Once the participants are through decorating their S and U cards, the professional tells them that he or she is going to give them scenarios or situations and they have to hold up their S card if they think it is safe or U card if they think it is unsafe.
5. The professional provides several scenarios and tries to match the scenarios to issues the group members need to improve.
6. Once the professional has finished, he or she can ask the group members if any of them want to share situations or scenarios and have the rest of the group respond with their safe or unsafe cards.

Processing and Application

At any point in this activity, the professional may need to stop and elaborate more on why a situation or behavior would be unsafe. Some children may have questions or may not understand why a situation would be unsafe. These questions should be addressed by the professional. Once the activity has been completed, the professional should ask the members if they have any questions about the activity or any questions about safe and unsafe behaviors.

Example Situations and Behaviors

- Crossing a street without looking for cars.
- Running across a parking lot.
- Getting into a car with a stranger.
- Wading out into a pond or lake.
- Running away from your parents in a store.
- Talking to someone you don't know online.
- Running away from home.
- Petting a strange dog or other animal.

Activity: Progressive Balloon Game

Social Skill Target Area(s)

Working together as a team and paying attention to another person

Level

Children

Materials

Balloons (one for every two participants)

Introduction

This activity can be done in pairs or in groups of four. It is a cooperative game where the participants must work together to keep a balloon in the air. The participants have to progress through four levels, with each level increasing in difficulty. Before implementing this activity, the professional should make sure none of the participants have a balloon allergy or a fear of balloons.

Instructions

1. The professional explains that they will be playing a game using balloons.
2. The professional divides the group into pairs and gives each pair a blown-up balloon.
3. The game has four levels and much like a video game, the pair must progress through each level and each level gets progressively more difficult. The pair must work together as a team to keep the balloon from hitting the floor.
4. The professional begins by telling the participants to hit the balloon back and forth any way they like and to keep it from hitting the floor (this level is not difficult, and most children will be able to do this very easily).
5. After a few minutes, the professional tells the participants to grab their balloons and now they will be progressing to the second level. In this level, the participants must take their dominant hand/arm and put it behind their back—they cannot use it. The participants begin hitting the balloon again with the objective to keep it from touching the ground.
6. After a few minutes, the professional tells the participants to grab their balloons and they have all progressed to the third level. In this

level, both hands/arms are put behind the back and cannot be used. The participants can use their feet, knees, and head. This level will be more challenging and some of the participants may have their balloons hit the ground. The professional should tell the children to pick their balloon up and keep going if it hits the ground.

7.   After a few minutes, the professional tells the participants to grab their balloons and they have all progressed to the final, fourth level. In this level the participants can only use their heads. They should try to hit the balloon back and forth 10 times without it touching the ground. After the participants have played this round for a few minutes, the professional can stop the activity.

8.   The professional can combine pairs and have one large group going through the progression using two or three balloons. This activity should be fun and not competitive. The professional will want to encourage the children to work tougher and support each other.

Processing and Application

Once the game has finished, the professional should ask the group how they felt about working with another person to keep the balloon in the air—was there anything that was difficult? Was there anything that seemed easy? The professional should ask the participants if they can think of other situations where they had to work with someone else to accomplish something. The professional can also ask participants to think about how they can get better at working together with others.

Activity: Midline Mirror Moves

Social Skill Target Area(s)

Connecting with others and focusing on another person

Level

Children

Materials

None

Introduction

Midline crossing moves have been demonstrated to cross the midline in the brain and help children improve focus, concentration, reduce anxiety, and increase regulation. This activity combines a common connection intervention, the mirroring game, with midline crossing moves. The benefits of this activity include helping children increase engagement and connection skills while working on improving regulation ability.

Instructions

1. The professional will have the group members stand up so that each member has some open space around them. The professional will stand in front of the group so each member can see the professional.
2. The professional will tell the group they must follow the professional's movements and mirror what the professional is doing.
3. The professional will then begin doing different movements and the participants will mirror. The professional should not move too fast and they will want to regularly create midline crossing moves. A midline crossing move is any movement where the body crosses such as a body hug or tapping elbow to alternate knee. Every move does not have to be a midline move but several of the movements should cross the midline.
4. The professional can decide how long he or she wants to continue the mirror midline activity.
5. Once the professional is finished, he or she can ask if there is anyone in the group who wants to lead the group in some more midline mirror moves. Any member who would like a turn should have the opportunity.
6. Another variation would be to have the group members pair up and each pair take turns doing the mirror midline moves to each other.

Processing and Application

This group activity can last as long as the professional and the members want to keep playing. Once the activity is over, the professional should process with the members if there was anything that felt uncomfortable or challenging about the activity. The professional may want to ask members how it felt to follow another person and, depending on the variations performed, what it felt like to do the activity as a whole group verses one on one with a partner.

Activity: Animal Feelings

Social Skill Target Area(s)

Emotion recognition, body language, and regulation ability

Level

Children

Materials

None

Introduction

Animal Feelings is a fun and interactive activity that can be silly while helping teach children about recognizing different feelings and what those feelings might look like. Many children with autism and developmental disorders struggle with understanding their emotions and how to express their emotions in a positive manner. This activity can be played repeatedly to help gain these skills.

Instructions

1. The professional instructs the children to stand around the room.
2. The professional explains that they are going to play a game called *Animal Feelings*.
3. The professional tells the children they will be naming an animal and putting a feeling with the animal. The children must act like that animal and express the feeling as they think that animal would. For example, the professional might say "Angry bear," and all the children then act like a bear who is feeling angry.
4. The professional allows the children to act like the feelings animal for around two minutes and then calls out a new animal feeling. The professional should go through several animal feelings.
5. Some examples of animal feelings include shy rabbit, excited fox, sad elephant, happy goat, worried chicken, proud lion, etc. The professional can make up several animal feelings and even change them up in the activity—there can be multiple happy or sad animals.
6. Once the professional has named a few animals, they can ask the group if any of the children want to lead in calling out animal feelings. Each child can have a turn if they want.

Processing and Application

One the activity has been completed, the professional should have the group sit in a circle and ask them how it felt to complete the activity. The professional will want to ask how it felt to try and identify different feelings and if that is something the children do well in their daily life. Some processing questions might include: Were you comfortable trying to express all the feelings, were some harder than others, did you notice anything about other children's feelings, and how do you think you could express your feelings in your daily life?

Activity: Volcano

Social Skill Target Area(s)

Emotional regulation and self-management ability

Level

Children

Materials

None

Introduction

Children with autism and developmental disorders often struggle with self-regulation ability and easily becoming dysregulated which can often lead to behavior meltdowns. This activity introduces children to understanding how dysregulation, frustration, and feelings of being upset can grow in a person and lead to a behavior explosion. It presents the concept in a fun and experiential method that can be replayed multiple times.

Instructions

1. The professional has the children stand around the room and explains to them that they will be playing an activity called *Volcano*.
2. The professional says he or she will guide the children through expressing how a volcano grows and explodes. They will be using their bodies to express the growing and exploding volcano.
3. The professional has the children get into a crouching position and grab their knees with their opposite hands. The professional tells the children they are volcanoes.
4. The professional then takes the child through a progression—the professional says:
5. "You are a volcano that is starting to get restless, start moving your body just a little bit. You are now getting more uncomfortable, move your body more and start to move your body out of the crouching position."
6. "Your volcano is now building more, you are getting more upset, move your body where you are now standing and your hands are to your side—continue to move your body around, shake a little bit."
7. "You are now getting pretty upset and getting ready to explode. Jump up and down a bit and move your body around more aggressively."

8. "You have now reached explosion! Jump around, move around the room, move quickly and wildly!" The professional should become more animated with this instruction. The children should stay in their explosion state for 20 seconds.
9. After around 20 seconds in the volcano explosion state, the professional should instruct the children to slow down and come back to a crouching position and repeat the whole process. The process should be completed a few times.

Processing and Application

After completing the volcano activity a few times, the professional should have all the children sit in a group and do some processing questions. The professional should begin by explaining that the volcano example illustrated how we can get dysregulated in our bodies and how the dysregulation builds to a behavior explosion. Some processing questions include: Have you noticed times when upset feelings have built up in you and then you "exploded"? What does it look like in your daily life when there is an explosion? What are some ideas to help you stop the build-up and not reach an explosion?

Activity: Sword Balloons

Social Skill Target Area(s)

Interacting (playing) with another person, competing (winning and losing), self-control, and regulation

Level

Children

Materials

Pool noodles (two) and balloons (one for every two participants)

Introduction

This activity uses pools noodles (as swords) and balloons to engage children in a fun and interactive activity which helps them learn to be more comfortable playing with another person in an organized game. It also works on helping children accept winning, losing, and general rule play. The sword and balloon action help increase self-control and regulation ability. Pool noodles are suggested for swords as they are soft and likely not to hurt if someone is accidently hit.

Instructions

1. The professional has the children get into pairs and gives each child a pool noodle sword and one balloon (blown up and tied off) for the pair. Each pair will need a bit of space from other pairs to ensure that children do not accidently hit other children with their swords.
2. The professional tells the children they are going to battle each other in a game of sword balloons.
3. The professional will say when to start and then the pair hit their balloon with their pool noodle swords. They are trying to hit the other person with the balloon. They cannot hit each other with the swords. The swords are used to hit the balloon toward their partner and to try and hit their partner with the balloon. They also cannot hit the balloon with their hands, they can only hit the balloon with their swords.
4. Often, children will accidently hit themselves with the balloon and this counts as a hit. The game can get very lively and should stay focused on having fun.
5. Once someone has been hit five times with the balloon, the game is over, and they can play another round.

6. The professional should monitor each pair to make sure children are not becoming frustrated, manage any disagreements, and keep the game fun and focused on skill development.

Processing and Application

The activity should be played for around 15 minutes and then the professional will have the children come together as a group for some process time. The professional should ask the group participants how it felt to play this game and interact with another person? What felt fun, easy, and challenging about it? The professional should ask the group's members to share about times in their daily life when they had to interact with or play with another person and how it went.

Activity: WRJMD

Social Skill Target Area(s)

Working (playing) as a group and regulation ability

Level

Children

Materials

None

Introduction

WRJMD stands for walk, run, jump, march, and dance. This activity is a fun group activity that provides the opportunity for children to participate together as a group and helps develop regulation skills. The acronym and the specific moves can be changed. Other options might include skipping, hopping, crawling, stomping, etc.

Instructions

1. The professional has the group participants stand somewhere in the room.
2. The professional says that he or she will play some fun music and then give the participants a specific move to be doing to the music. This activity does not require music. If the professional does not have access to music or if there are participants who have a music sensitivity, music does not need to be played.
3. The professional will change the move after about two minutes.
4. Using the WRJMD acronym, the professional will start by asking the participants to walk around the room. After about two minutes, the professional will switch to run around the room, after two minutes switch to jump around the room, then march, and lastly dance around the room.
5. Once the activity has been completed, the professional can take the participants through the activity again playing a different song.

Processing and Application

This activity should not last longer than 20 minutes. Once it has been completed, the professional should have the group members come together for processing. The professional should ask the members how it felt to participate in this activity with each other. Some additional processing questions might include: Have you ever participated in a fun group activity in your daily life, and how did it go? Also, the professional can ask the participants what felt good and not so good completing the activity and process through their responses.

Activity: Group Machine

Social Skill Target Area(s)

Completing a task with a group, teamwork, engagement, and communication

Level

Children

Materials

None

Introduction

Group Machine gives participants the opportunity to work together as a group and accomplish a task. The process is designed to be fun and engaging and allow the children to feel empowered in working together, communicating and achieving a task. Many children with autism struggle in group formats, especially working with a group to complete a task. *Group Machine* is a successful activity to help children with autism become more competent in these skills.

Instructions

1. The professional shares with the participants that the group is going to be working together to complete a task. If you are seeing a large group (8–10 participants), you may want to create two groups instead of one large group for this activity.
2. The professional explains that the group is going to create a machine using their bodies. Each person in the group will be a part of the machine that is created. The professional should present the activity in a fun and playful way encouraging the group to have fun with the activity.
3. The group must decide what machine they are creating and what part of the machine each person will be.
4. The machine should have a name and a purpose.
5. The group must also design how each part of the machine (each person) connects physically together.
6. Once the group has finished their design, they will present the machine to the professional. One person will introduce the machine (name and what it is for), then each person will connect to each other one at a time and say what part of the machine they are.

7. This is a higher-level activity for group members. It will challenge many of their social skill deficits. The professional should monitor the process and assist the group if needed. The professional should monitor for proper communication, working together, each person contributing, and making sure the members are not becoming too anxious or dysregulated by the activity.

Processing and Application

Once the group has finished presenting their design, the professional asks the group to sit in a circle for some processing time. The professional should ask the participants what it felt like to work together as a group to create the machine. Additional processing questions could include: What part was hard for you? What part was easy? Have you ever worked with a group before to accomplish a task? The professional should share any observations they had watching the group process and ask any questions they might have about what they observed.

Activity: Backward Moves

Social Skill Target Area(s)

Following instructions, participating in an activity with a group, regulation ability

Level

Children

Materials

None

Introduction

This activity provides a fun and interactive game that the whole group plays together. The professional facilitates a series of moves that the group members must complete backwards. The moves the professional presents include walking, hopping, moving in slow motion, swimming, dancing, crawling, etc. all done backwards. Participants must navigate around each other and follow instructions presented by the professional. This activity also helps improve regulation ability.

Instructions

1. The professional has the group members stand around the room.
2. The professional explains that they are going to complete a group activity where the professional will call out different moves to do and the participants must do the moves backward.
3. The professional should be sure to explain that participants should be aware of each other and try to avoid running into each other.
4. The professional begins by telling the participants to walk around the room backward. After one to two minutes, the professional says to hop backwards around the room. After about two minutes, the professional says to walk quickly backwards, then act like you are swimming backward, then move in slow motion, then dance, and lastly crawl backward. The professional can add additional moves if they would like.
5. It's also fun to add having the group try to pronounce different words backward, such as think of how to say the word "play" backward, then give a countdown and have all the group members try to pronounce the word backward in unison.

Processing and Application

Once the activity has been played, the professional can have some processing time with the group. The professional can begin by asking the members how it felt to play the activity together and if there was anything that was challenging. The professional can also ask the members what their experience has been playing with peers in a group activity or game. The professional will also want to share any observations they had watching the group interaction.

SOCIAL SKILLS INTERVENTIONS FOR ADOLESCENTS

Activity: Bubble Tag

Social Skill Target Area(s)

Cooperation, working together as a group, listening, and communicating

Level

Adolescents

Materials

Bubbles (one bottle for every member of the group)

Introduction

This activity involves the whole group playing together. Bubbles are used to play a game of tag and throughout the course of the game, each child is working on a team trying to achieve a common goal. It is most helpful to play this game in a small to medium size space with some boundaries. This activity is also very fun and lively. Once the game has been played, it can be repeated several times.

Instructions

1. The professional tells the group they are going to play a game of tag using bubbles.
2. The professional explains that there will be two participants who will be given bubbles and they are the taggers. They must tag other group members by blowing bubbles and touching the other participants with bubbles (they do not tag or touch them with their hands).
3. The professional establishes what the boundaries are of the room (where participants can move around).
4. The professional gives each tagger a bottle of bubbles and tells the group they can begin. If someone gets touched by any bubble, they then get a bottle of bubbles and join the taggers trying to get the rest of the group.
5. This continues until everyone in the group has been tagged.
6. The professional can participate and start out being a tagger.
7. This activity usually does not take long to complete. It can be repeated several times.

Processing and Application

This is a whole group activity and regardless of what is happening, each child is always part of a group with a common purpose. It provides a fun and engaging way for the group to play together and experience being together in a social game. Once the activity has been completed, the professional should ask the group members how it felt to participate in the game. The professional should ask the participants to share about any part of the activity that felt uncomfortable or challenging.

Activity: Keep It Going

Social Skill Target Area(s)

Cooperation, completing a group task, and joint attention

Level

Adolescents

Materials

White piece of paper (one for every two participants) and pencils

Introduction

This activity is completed in pairs and focuses on playing and completing a task together. As the name implies, the activity can be played until the participants are no longer interested. It does require drawing, but it is not necessary to be a "good" drawer to participate in the activity. Professionals will want to stress this point to the group members before beginning the activity.

Instructions

1. The professional explains that the group will be completing an activity by working in pairs.
2. The professional should divide the group members into pairs and the professional can participate if needed.
3. The professional gives each pair a white piece of paper and each person gets a pencil.
4. The professional states that one person will start and draws a simple squiggle or line somewhere on the piece of paper. The other person then must take the squiggle or line and turn it into a picture of something.
5. The pictures are typically simple and sometime silly. The drawing does not have to be elaborate or even accurate.
6. Once the person is finished turning the squiggle into a picture of something, the person draws a squiggle or line somewhere on the paper and then the other person has to turn that squiggle or line into a picture of something. This keeps going back and forth until the participants are no longer interested in playing.
7. Typically, a white piece of paper will be full of eight to ten drawings by the time the activity ends.

Processing and Application

When it seems like the participants are no longer interested in keeping the drawing activity going, the professional can end the activity. The professional will want to process with the group what it felt like to work and play with another person in this capacity—what was challenging and what felt okay? If there is time, the professional could have the group members rotate playing this activity with each member of the group to create different social experiences.

Activity: Circle Picture (Turner-Bumberry, 2019)

Social Skill Target Area(s)

Cooperation, working in a group, following directions, and taking turns

Level

Adolescents

Materials

Large piece of paper, pencils, colored pencils, compass or circle templates (circle templates can be found at art supply stores)

Introduction

This activity allows group members to create art together but challenges them by having to take turns and creating only one piece of artwork. Circles can be relaxing shapes to draw which may help individuals while working within the group.

Instructions

1. The professional gives each group member a pencil. The group members sit in a circle with a large piece of paper in the center.
2. The professional starts by taking a compass or a circle template and drawing one circle anywhere on the paper. The professional then explains that each group member will get to do the same. They also explain that circles can overlap each other and be placed anywhere on the paper.
3. The paper is passed clockwise with each group member choosing a circle size and drawing a circle on the paper. Paper can continue to be passed around to where each group member gets two or three turns drawing a circle.
4. When the drawing is complete, the professional can have the group members color in the circles, or parts of the circles since there may be overlapping. The professional should be more directive with this part of the activity if they feel the group members cannot complete this activity successfully (example: assigning each group member part of the page to color).

Processing and Application

The professional may ask the group questions at the end of this activity including: How did it feel creating circles the first time/second time/third time? Was it easier or more difficult the second/third time? Explain why? What did you enjoy about this shared artwork? What was a challenge? Did the artwork turn out how you thought it would? How is working in a group different than working alone? What skills did you need to practice to make this activity successful? Are there other times/places/ activities where you have to work in a group? How can you use the skills you practiced here in those situations?

Activity: Color by Number Picture (Turner-Bumberry, 2019)

Social Skill Target Area(s)

Cooperating with peers, taking turns, and following instructions

Level

Adolescents

Materials

Have a simple mandala printed. The professional should lightly place a number into each part of the mandala; the number should correspond to the total number of group members. This activity also needs a bucket of crayons.

Introduction

This is an artistic activity that is also low pressure for group members. The mandala is already drawn, so it simply needs to be colored in. This activity allows group members to color using their favorite color, but also challenges them to accept the favorite colors of other group members. There is an additional challenge to take turns and follow the directions.

Instructions

1. The professional has each group member pick their favorite color from a bucket of crayons.
2. The professional then assigns each group member a number from one to ___ (largest number is total number of group members).
3. The professional has the group members sit in a circle and places the mandala in the center of the circle. The professional shows them how the mandala has numbers on it. The professional explains that group member number one will color all of the spaces with a one inside with their particular color.
4. This continues with group member two, three, four, etc. coloring in their spaces in the mandala that has their number inside. The activity is complete when the mandala is colored by all group members.

Processing and Application

Once the activity has been completed, the professional may ask the group questions which might include: While looking at the completed mandala what are your thoughts/feelings about it? Would this picture have looked differently if you would have chosen the colors yourself? Completed the activity yourself? How did it feel to share in this activity? What do you think about sharing responsibilities? What are other activities where you have to take turns and share responsibilities? Why is this an important skill for you to practice?

Activity: Feelings Collage (Turner-Bumberry, 2019)

Social Skill Target Area(s)

Expressing and sharing feelings, listening to feelings of others, following instructions, and giving compliments

Level

Adolescents

Materials

One sheet of paper for each group member, various magazines, scissors, glue, and markers

Introduction

This activity will allow group members to further explore one feeling of their choosing. Pictures instead of words will be used to describe this feeling. Group members will share their collages and give compliments to the collages of the other group members.

Instructions

1. The professional will explain to group members that each person will need to choose a feeling and not share with the other members which feeling they chose (the group can decide if they are okay with the chance that the same feeling is chosen by several group members or not. If not, each group member can whisper in the professional's ear what they chose, and he or she can let them know if that feeling was chosen already).
2. The professional will give each group member a sheet of paper and magazines will be available for all. The professional will instruct group members to go through the magazines and tear/cut out any pictures that remind them of their chosen feeling.
3. Once pictures are chosen, the group members will each glue their pictures onto their pieces of paper, creating a collage.
4. When completed, group members can each share their collage, expressing why they chose the pictures, or a feeling guessing game can be played based on the context of the pictures.
5. Group members will each give a compliment to the individual that is presenting, focusing on pictures chosen, presentation, expression of feelings, etc.

Processing and Application

Once every group member has shared, the professional may ask the group additional processing questions such as: Was it easier or harder to use pictures to describe your feeling? Did you notice any similarities between your chosen pictures and the pictures of other group members? Did any group member share something that you can relate to? How can we use pictures at home/school/etc. to let people know how we're feeling?

Activity: Act As If (Turner-Bumberry, 2019)

Social Skill Target Area(s)

Handling anxiety and practicing body awareness

Level

Adolescents

Materials

None

Introduction

In therapeutic sessions, we may forget at times to focus on wellness rather than deficits. With this activity we discuss what it may look like to actually feel the opposite of negative feelings, and then use movement to show the positive feelings. This can help group members feel their bodies' responding to positive emotions. They can then take one small action of this expression to practice when feeling dysregulated.

Instructions

1. The professional brainstorms with group members about what their body feels like when anxious (examples include shaking, head down, mumbling, shoulders hunched, etc.).
2. The professional mimics the suggestions by moving their body how group members have described.
3. The professional then brainstorms with group members what opposite movements would look like (examples include head up, speaking clearly, standing up straight, smiling, etc.).
4. The professional mimics the suggestions by moving their body how group members have described, then invites other group members to walk around the room "as if" they are not anxious.

Processing and Application

The professional should process with the group members once the activity has been completed. Some sample processing questions include: How did it feel to walk around the room "as if" you had no anxiety? What is one of the movements you can try to start doing when feeling anxious? Where could moving "as if" you had no anxiety be helpful?

Activity: Hand Jive

Social Skill Target Area(s)

Working in a group, cooperation, and understanding appropriate social norms

Level

Adolescents

Materials

None

Introduction

This is a fun way for each group member to use an appropriate hand movement to create a group hand jive. The hand jive can easily be used for an opening or closing transition for subsequent groups. The professional should be prepared for possible inappropriate gestures to be mentioned and if this happens, calmly explain that the gesture would be inappropriate in a social setting. Other group members can also help explain what could happen if the inappropriate gesture were displayed in various social settings.

Instructions

1. The professional brainstorms with group members the multiple friendly gestures our hands can do that are appropriate in social settings (examples include waving, high fiving, thumbs up, etc.).
2. Each group member chooses the friendly hand gesture that they want to use for the hand jive. It can be a real or made up gesture, as long as it would not be seen as inappropriate in social settings.
3. Once each group member has chosen a hand gesture, the hand jive is created using each gesture from each group member in a continuous movement.
4. Hand jive is practiced multiple times, possibly written down to remember, and can accompany music.

Processing and Application

Once the hand jive activity has been done a few times, the professional may ask the group some processing questions such as: How can friendly gestures be helpful in social settings? How can unfriendly gestures be unhelpful in social settings? This activity can assist in opening a discussion about body language—understanding other people's body language and how we communicate through our own body language.

Activity: I Spy

Social Skill Target Area(s)

Recognizing the emotions of others and communicating feelings to others

Level

Adolescents

Materials

A blanket large enough for all group members to sit on

Introduction

I Spy is an excellent intervention to teach to parents for their group sessions. It can also be done with the professional who has access to public areas for viewing. It is important for the parent or professional to have the group members sitting at a distance from the public so as not to be overheard while practicing emotion recognition. It is also advisable for the professional or parent to first model how the game is played for greater understanding. Group members may also need to be reminded to not point or yell out during this game; it's strictly a game within the group.

Instructions

1. The professional or parent brings group members to a public place and has them sit on a blanket an appropriate distance from other people and activity (example places include parks, outdoor plazas, etc.).
2. The professional or parent states they are going to play the game *I Spy*. The group members will observe the people around them and propose a feeling they believe a person or other people are feeling. When they believe they have enough context, they can call out "I spy someone who is feeling _____."
3. Once a group member has called this out, other group members guess which person or people the individual has noticed. Once the correct person has been chosen, group members discuss clues they had to help them guess the feeling.
4. This activity can be played for several minutes, ideally allowing time for each group member to share something they notice.

Processing and Application

Once the activity has been completed, the professional may ask the group questions for further processing. Some example questions include: What did you notice while playing this game? Why do you think we needed to sit away from the public while playing this group? What would have been inappropriate to do while playing this game? What are clues we noticed about people who were (happy, mad, sad, etc.)? How can this game help you at (school, home, grocery store, etc.)?

Activity: What to Say Scripts

Social Skill Target Area(s)

Discussing emotions, sharing with a group, and handling difficult situations

Level

Adolescents

Materials

Index cards and pencils

Introduction

Adolescents with ASD not only struggle with social skills, but also with emotion regulation. When angered by other peers, they often revert to less effective coping methods, such as crying, screaming, hitting themselves, etc. Writing a short script that can be practiced with group members who are struggling socially can provide an effective means for ensuring success when these difficult situations occur.

Instructions

1. The professional begins by describing how all of us struggle with what to say when someone upsets us. Having a short phrase written and practiced can often be a useful tool in helping us stay calm when angered (the professional may wish to share an example to help lessen the discomfort with sharing).
2. The professional asks the group member to share something that has been said to them which has made them upset. If the group seems less inclined to share personal anecdotes, the professional can instead ask what things might make adolescents their age upset.
3. Once a group member has spoken, the professional asks other group members to share ideas of a brief phrase that may be an effective coping statement for that situation. The professional should be ready to give an example to help with the group discussion, or even have common coping phrases/mantras available for viewing.
4. The group member who shared first then chooses one phrase they wish to use as their coping statement and writes it on their index card. Steps 2–4 continue until every group member has completed this activity.
5. The remaining session time is spent with the group members getting into pairs and practicing using their coping statements. They may

choose to practice the statement without the other group member saying the hurtful phrase if it causes too much dysregulation, however the goal is for the participants to be able to hear the statement in practice to help gain confidence with their response.

6. The professional should encourage this to be practiced multiple times at home, so the group members are prepared if/when they encounter the hurtful statement.

Processing and Application

The professional may provide some processing directives at the end of this activity including: Describe the bravery it took for you to share with the group something that upsets you. Discuss the feelings you felt when recounting the statement that upset you. Discuss the feelings you felt when the other group members were helping you with helpful coping statements.

Activity: Safe Zones

Social Skill Target Area(s)

Identifying places to feel safe, recognizing need for strategies, and working in a group

Level

Adolescents

Materials

Graph paper, pencils, small red, yellow, and green dot stickers

Introduction

There are many places where adolescents with autism may feel overwhelmed and anxious. Discussing this, while also coming up with safe zones within these places can empower clients to feel more comfortable when being in these places. Group members will also discover that they are not alone in feeling this dysregulation which may normalize their feelings of anxiety.

Instructions

1. The professional begins by expressing how certain places can make us feel anxious. Examples might include school, grocery stores, church, etc.
2. The professional invites the group members to share a place that makes them feel anxious, uncomfortable, or dysregulated.
3. Once group members share, the professional hands each adolescent a piece of graph paper and a pencil. The professional invites the group members to each draw a simple floor plan of the place that causes anxiety. The professional may have a simple sketch drawn already for reference. Listing the rooms and areas within the place would also be helpful for the group members to do.
4. Once completed, the professional asks each group member to look at their drawings and think about where within this place it may be possible to feel calmer or more regulated? Where within this place may they be able to use their coping skills in a safer, acceptable, more private space? The professional hands each group member a sheet containing green, yellow, and red stickers dots The professional has the members mark safe places with a green dot (consider a floorplan of a school for example, green spaces may include special education room, nurse's office, counselor's office, etc.).

5. The professional then has the group members mark with a red dot those spaces within the floor plan where it would not feel safe, acceptable or private to calm down and regulate (using the school example, red spaces may include music room, gym, playground).

6. The professional then has the group members mark with a yellow dot those spaces within the floor plan where they are not sure if it would feel safe, acceptable or private to calm down and regulate. They would need to talk to an adult and explore if this space was an option. These areas would be marked with a yellow dot (using the school example, yellow spaces may include a classroom, the office, etc.).

7. Each group member can share and discuss their floorplans with the rest of the group.

Processing and Application

The professional may ask the group processing questions at the end of this activity. A lot of processing has occurred during this activity, so this part may be brief, and only focus on a plan of how they can incorporate their floorplan into action.

Activity: Oops and Ouch

Social Skill Target Area(s)

Expressing feelings and understanding others' point of view

Level

Adolescents

Materials

Two index cards for each group member, one with the word "Oops!" on it; one with the word "Ouch!" on it; the "Oops!" script and "Ouch!" script (example scripts at the end of this activity description)

Introduction

Often adolescents on the ASD are very honest and can hurt others' feelings with this honesty. They can also feel hurt by what others say to them but be unable to express these hurt feelings. This activity helps group members begin to recognize when they may be hurting someone's feelings and express when their own feelings are being hurt. This activity is excellent for practicing at home, and the professional may want to give group members extra index cards for the entire family to use.

Instructions

1. The professional gives each group member two index cards, one card has the word "Oops!" on it; the other has the word "Ouch!" on it.
2. The professional begins dialogue by discussing how sometimes we may say something that hurts someone's feelings and not even know it. The professional may give an example and then invite other group members to share examples.
3. The professional next begins discussion on how sometimes we may have our feelings hurt and not be sure how to let that person know. They may give an example and then invite other group members to share examples.
4. The professional then explains that the "Oops!" and "Ouch!" cards are going to help them begin to explore how to let people know that their feelings have been hurt as well as how they may have hurt other's feelings.
5. The professional explains the "Oops!" card is used whenever a person realizes they may have said something insulting. When this happens, the person talking should stop, hold up the card, and say

"Oops!" This gives the other person a chance to share if their feelings were hurt, or if they were not.

6. The professional then explains the "Ouch!" card is used whenever a person is hurt by what someone has said to them. When this happens, the person holds up the card and says "Ouch!" This gives the talker a chance to stop talking, ask for clarification, and apologize if needed.

7. The professional first has two group members read the "Oops!" script aloud. The professional tells the other group members to hold up the "Oops!" card and say "Oops!" whenever they feel one of the characters may be saying something hurtful or inappropriate. Whenever any group member does this, the professional should stop the reading and have a discussion on which character may have been inappropriate, what they said that was inappropriate, and what they could have possibly said instead.

8. The professional then has two other group members read the "Ouch!" script aloud. The professional tells the other group members to hold up the "Ouch!" card and say "Ouch!" whenever they feel one of the characters may have hurt feelings. Whenever any group member does this, the professional should stop the reading and have a discussion on which character may have hurt feelings, what was said that made his feelings hurt, and what he could possibly say to the other character.

Processing and Application

The professional may ask the group questions at the end of this activity including: Can we think of an example where something we said may have hurt someone else's feelings? How can we start noticing this, so we aren't hurting people's feelings? Can we think of an example where something that was said to us hurt our feelings? How can we start letting people know they have hurt our feelings? Did all of us agree on what were "Oops!" statements and what were "Ouch!" statements when we heard the stories? What could that be telling us about each other?

Sample "Oops" Script

(Group members are listening for when the speaker may need to stop what they are saying because they may be speaking hurtfully.)

Jamie: Hi Jackie, how are you?
Jackie: I'm doing great Jamie!
Jamie: Do you want to play basketball with me? We can take turns trying to throw the ball into the net.
Jackie: Sounds great, let's do it!
Jamie: I'll throw the ball first, because I'm much better than you. You can watch me and then learn how to be better.

Jackie:	Oh.
Jamie:	Oh man, I missed it, the ball didn't go in like I thought!
Jackie:	Ha! Ha! You're not as good as you think!
Jamie:	I guess not!
Jackie:	Woo hoo! I got that one in! Yes!
Jamie:	Nice job!
Jackie:	Thanks!
Jamie:	I'm surprised you got it in, you're usually really bad at this.
Jackie:	Am I?
Jamie:	Yes, I watched you play, and you are usually terrible at basketball.
Jackie:	Well, at least I am a genius at math where you are really, really bad at multiplication.
Jamie:	Oh, that's my mom calling me, I better go inside! See you later Jackie!
Jackie:	See you later Jamie!

Sample "Ouch!" Script

(Group members are listening for when the listener may be feeling hurt because of what is being said to them).

Antwan:	Hi Marcus, what are you doing right now?
Marcus:	What does it look like I'm doing?
Antwan:	I don't know, that's why I asked.
Marcus:	I'm trying to build a Lego tower, only using yellow Legos.
Antwan:	That's really dumb, I hate the color yellow.
Marcus:	Whatever, Antwan. Do you want to help me build it?
Antwan:	Sure, but do I have to only use yellow Legos?
Marcus:	No, just pick your favorite color and we can have a two-color tower.
Antwan:	O.K.
Marcus:	What are you doing? That looks horrible!
Antwan:	I'm just adding a landing over here, I think it looks cool.
Marcus:	I guess that's ok.
Antwan:	It's definitely o.k. because your tower was boring and plain, so I needed to make it look better.
Marcus:	Well it doesn't look better, it looks worse, so you aren't helpful at all.
Antwan:	I'm just going to build my own tower next to yours.
Marcus:	That's a good idea, then we can have two towers!
Antwan:	Maybe later we can build a parking lot with some cars.
Marcus:	Maybe, but let's just do our towers right now.

Activity: Architects

Social Skill Target Area(s)

Working together, compromising, and taking turns

Level

Adolescents

Materials

Duct tape, newspaper, yarn, straws, and scissors

Introduction

This activity can be completed with all of the group members working together or by dividing the group members into teams of two or three. This is up to the professional based on how well the group members can work in teams. *Architects* is a fun way to work on team building while creating a structure of their choice. Having free reign as a team on deciding what to create can cause some differences of opinion. This gives the group members opportunity to practice the skills of compromise and taking turns. The professional may need to give reminders of the importance of working as a team when completing this activity.

Instructions

1. The professional gives group members a roll of duct tape, a ball of yarn, some newspaper, straws, and scissors (if dividing the group into smaller teams, each team will need these items).
2. The professional explains that the team will create whatever structure they want only using these four items (the scissors are used for cutting only).
3. The professional tells the group to first discuss with each other possible items to build. Once the group comes to a consensus on what should be built, they can then start the construction.
4. The professional gives the group 20 minutes to create their structure, monitoring the group for turn taking, compromise, and teamwork.

Processing and Application

Once the group members are finished creating their structure. The professional can make comments about what he or she observed and ask the group some processing questions. Some example processing questions include: What was easy about working as a team? What was difficult about working as a team? Did the structure turn out as you thought it would—how so or not? Did you have to compromise in the group—how so? What were the benefits about working as a team to complete this activity?

Activity: Communication Blocks

Social Skill Target Area(s)

Communication, listening, following instructions, working together to complete a task, and perspective taking

Level

Adolescents

Materials

Two matching sets of blocks or Legos

Introduction

This activity is designed to help adolescents work on improving their ability to communicate and listen effectively when interacting with another person. It also develops perspective taking—working on theory of mind deficits. The participants work in pairs while the professional observes and can better assess the skill deficits the adolescents might be struggling with. Blocks, Legos, or pictures can be used in this activity and it can be repeated many times for additional skill work. Wood or foam blocks can be used, Legos, or a picture can be drawn, and the other person given instructions on drawing the same picture. This activity will highlight communication skills and deficits and is a good activity to do early in the group meetings and possibly again toward the end of the group meetings to note improvements in skill development.

Instructions

1. The professional tells the participants they are going to be working on an activity called communication blocks (or Legos, or pictures). The professional has the group members get into pairs sitting with their backs to each other.
2. The professional gives both members in the pair a matching set of blocks—so each person has the same blocks in front of them.
3. One person in the pair is designated the instructor and the other is designated the listener (builder). The instructor builds something with their blocks. Once they are finished, they are going to tell the listener to build the same thing—giving them instructions on exactly what to build without being able to see what the instructor built (remember their backs are to each other the whole time). The

instructor tries to give detailed instructions and the listener can ask questions with the goal being that both builds come out identical.

4. Once the pair feel like they are finished, they can turn around and see what each other built.
5. If there is time, the activity can be repeated with the pair switching roles.
6. While the activity is being done, the professional should be walking around the room and observing each pair in the process. The professional might want to take notes on communication style, listening skills, frustration tolerance, and any other things they may notice and want to mention during the processing time.

Processing and Application

Once everyone has finished, they can stay in their pairs for processing time. Each pair can share how their builds came out. The professional should ask the group how it felt to be in this process, what was challenging and if anything felt easy. The professional should also address any notes they took while observing each pair in the building process. This is a good time to talk about strengths observed and suggestions for skills that need to be improved. If there is time, the activity can be repeated with a focus on improving the skills that need strengthen or the activity can be implemented again in a later group meeting.

Activity: Follow the Leader

Social Skill Target Area(s)

Following instructions, listening, attention, and self-regulation

Level

Adolescents

Materials

None

Introduction

Follow the Leader is a fun and silly activity that helps adolescents adhere to social rules, follow instructions, and work on paying attention. It is completed as a whole group exercise and can have many elements added to the activity. It does require some space to move around—it would be challenging to complete this activity in a small room. Because it is a highly playful activity, it could be implemented in an early group session to help participants feel more relaxed.

Instructions

1. The professional explains they will be doing an activity called *Follow the Leader*.
2. The professional has all the members stand up and get into a line, one behind the other but giving each other some space.
3. The professional explains they will be at the front of the line and will lead the line around the room while giving out instructions for what the line needs to do. The professional will make different moves or actions and the rest of the line must mimic the professional. For example, the professional will start walking and everyone else starts walking (in line) and then the professional might start waving their hands in the air while they are walking—the line would start waving their hands in the air while walking. Anything the professional does, the rest of the line does, and the professional keeps the line walking around the room while doing different moves.
4. Some examples of moves to do in the line include waving hands in the air, making a sound, clapping hands, stomping feet, doing a right or left leg kick out, flapping hands, putting hands on top of your head, hopping, laughing, walking on tippy toes, dancing, act like you are a plane, spin around, act like you are playing a video game, act like

you are driving a car, etc. Anything the professional can think of, they can do. It's important to keep it fun and silly so the participants can enjoy the experience.

5. After the professional has led the line a few minutes, the professional should ask if any of the participants want to be the leader. The professional should let each of the members be the leader if they want, but no one should be forced to be the leader if they are uncomfortable.

Processing and Application

Once the activity has been completed (which should be no longer than 15–20 minutes), the professional has the group sit in a circle for processing time. The professional should ask the members how it felt to participate in this activity. Additional processing questions might include: What was your favorite part of this activity? Was there anything you did not like or felt uncomfortable? If you were a leader, how did it feel to be the leader?

Activity: Play-Doh Relax

Social Skill Target Area(s)

Following instructions, listening, regulation, and relaxation

Level

Adolescents

Materials

Play-Doh (one for each participant)

Introduction

This activity simultaneously works on social skills such as following instructions, listening, completing a task sequence while working on interpersonal skills such as regulation, coping skills, and relaxation. Each participant has their own Play-Doh (it is recommended to have the normal size not the small size bottles). If any members have a sensitivity to Play-Doh, then this activity would not be implemented.

Instructions

1. The professional passes out a Play-Doh to each group members. If the professional has several colors, the participants can choose their own color.
2. The professional explains they are doing to take the group though a series of activities they will be doing with the Play-Doh.
3. The group's members can take out their Play-Doh and begin to manipulate it in their hands.
4. The professional then begins to provide instructions for what to do with the Play-Doh. The following guide can be used, or the professional can create their own version.

   a. Roll the Play-Doh into a ball in your hands.
   b. Squeeze the Play-Doh in your left hand.
   c. Roll the Play-Doh into a snake between your hands.
   d. Cut or pinch the Play-Doh off into seven pieces.
   e. Roll the Play-Doh into a ball between your hands.
   f. Squeeze the Play-Doh in your right hand.
   g. Using your palms, smash the Play-Doh into a thin layer.
   h. Make a fist with your left hand, take the Play-Doh and cover your fist, pressing it down to mold it around your left-hand fist.

i.   Do the same thing to your right hand.
j.   Finish playing with the Play-Doh as you like or turn it into anything you want.

Processing and Application

Each of the steps in the Play-Doh sequence should last around two minutes. The professional can add steps and actions. The ending allows the participants two minutes to play with the Play-Doh however they like. Once the activity has been completed, the professional should ask the participants some processing questions, such as: How did it feel to complete this activity? Did you feel relaxed doing this activity? Was there any step that you enjoyed more than the others? Was there any step that you did not like? The professional should also discuss completing this activity or a version of this activity at home or other places when the members might feel anxious, worried, or upset. The professional can ask the members if they can think of a situation where they might use the activity to help them in their daily life.

Activity: Magazine Minute (social group version)

Social Skill Target Area(s)

Noticing others, understanding social context, and body language

Level

Adolescents

Materials

A variety of magazines

Introduction

This activity can work on a variety of social skills and provides the opportunity to discuss several different social situations. The professional will need to have several magazines available to use with this activity. The professional should look through each magazine to make sure there is no inappropriate content in the magazines. *Magazine Minute* can be played several times and with different instructions. Some examples are provided in the instructions section, but the professional may want to implement their own versions.

Instructions

1. The professional has several magazines on a table (the magazines should have examples through stories and/or advertisements of people in different situations or people in general).
2. The professional explains that each member can take a couple of magazines, and when the professional says, "Go," the participants will have one minute to find an example of a person or people in the magazine that are in some type of social situation.
3. Once the minute is up, each member will share the picture they found and talk about what social situation they believe is happening. They can share what they think the situation is, how people are reacting, feeling, or anything they want to say about what is happening socially.
4. The professional can help any member that is struggling to identify what is happening socially and other group members can add what they think is happening in other members pictures.
5. The professional should then complete the process a couple more times as time permits.

Processing and Application

Once the activity has finished, the professional can have a processing time with the members. Some suggested processing questions include: How did it feel completing this activity? What felt challenging to you and what felt easy? Did you find pictures that seemed confusing or that you did not understand what was happening? How does this apply to your daily life when you see people in social situations? This activity can prompt a good discussion about the members daily life and struggles in social situations in which they do not understand what is happening or feel challenged in participating.

Activity: Wall Draw

Social Skill Target Area(s)

Completing a task together, teamwork, cooperation, paying attention to another person, and communication skills

Level

Adolescents

Materials

Large piece of paper, tape, and markers

Introduction

Wall Draw is a whole group activity. If the social skills group has a large number of members (8–10), this activity should be divided into two groups. This activity gives the group members an opportunity to work together as a team to complete a task. Often, adolescents with autism struggle in peer groups especially when asked to work in a group setting to accomplish something. *Wall Draw* is a fun and relaxed way to develop skills related to participating in a group. The professional will want to observe each group member and possibly take notes on skill strengths and struggles.

Instructions

1. The professional explains to the group they will be drawing a picture together. The professional makes sure to state that drawing skills are not necessary to complete this task and the objective is fun—not creating a great drawing.
2. The professional hangs a large piece of paper on the wall or lays it on a table.
3. The professional gives each member a different color marker.
4. The professional decides on the drawing order giving each participate a number indicating when they will draw on the paper.
5. The professional explains that each member will go in number order to the paper and draw something. Each member will have 20 seconds to draw. When their 20 seconds are up, the next person will go for 20 seconds and draw on the paper. This will continue until each member has drawn on the paper twice. The group members can talk and decide on a unified picture to draw or they can randomly add to

the picture. This will be something the group needs to decide. The professional can provide guidance if needed.

6. Once the picture has been completed, the members can look at the finished product and notice each person's contribution (remember each person will have their own color of marker).

7. All the members can then sign the picture they have created together.

Processing and Application

Once the picture has been completed, the professional asks the group members some processing questions, such as: What did it feel like to complete this picture together? Was it easy to work together or difficult? What was the easiest part and hardest part for you? Do you think it would have felt better to draw your own picture? The professional can also share any observations they noted while the members were completing the picture. The professional can also ask the members about times in their daily life when they had to work with a group and what was the experience like.

Activity: Make a Monster

Social Skill Target Area(s)

Teamwork, communication skills, listening, frustration tolerance, and trust

Level

Adolescents

Materials

Piece of paper, marker, scissors, and a blindfold (handkerchief or scarf)

Introduction

Many adolescents with autism struggle interacting with their peers, especially in-person conversation and communication of any kind. This activity helps children develop communication skills as well as teamwork skills through a fun and engaging game. Further skill development includes listening skills and managing frustration tolerance. The professional will do some pre-meeting set up with this activity. The professional will draw an outline of a monster on a piece of paper (it should be a large outline). The professional will then cut the monster into puzzle pieces (the number of pieces should match the number of group members). The professional will want to have this ready prior to the group meeting.

Instructions

1. The professional will explain to the group they will be completing an activity called *Make a Monster*.
2. The professional will give each member a piece of the monster puzzle and explain to the participants that these are pieces of a monster outline.
3. The group must work together to complete the puzzle (make the monster).
4. Each member will take a turn placing their pieces on the table to try and connect to other members pieces and complete the puzzle. But the person who is putting their piece in play will be blindfolded and the rest of the group must communicate to that person where to place their puzzle piece.
5. For example, each member takes a turn placing their piece. The person who is going must be blindfolded with a handkerchief or a scarf. The rest of the group guides that person to where they place their

piece. They then take off their blindfold and it is given to the person who goes next. This continues until all the pieces have been placed correctly and the monster has been made.

6. The professional should be observing the interaction among the group members, specifically noting communication strengths and deficits.

Processing and Application

Once the puzzle has been completed, the professional processes the activity with the group. Some suggested processing questions include: How did you feel completing this activity? What was challenging and what was easy? How did it feel to be blindfolded and having to rely on the group members to help you? What do you feel like you learned from completing this activity? The professional should also share any observations they made while watching the group complete the activity.

8   Conclusion

Ryan entered his first AutPlay social skills group along with five other preadolescent boys all diagnosed with Asperger's Syndrome. Ryan's social experiences with peers included a history of confusion and rejection. Ryan was hesitant to be in a group with several other peers and his early group sessions were a combination of withdrawn behavior and being overly assertive which often presented as annoying. After a few meetings, Ryan began to feel comfortable; he began to see the group as a safe place and his peers as possibilities for friendships. He began to think that this peer group was not the same as peer interactions of the past. No one in the group was rejecting him and they were accepting him, even when he displayed overly assertive behavior.

Session by session, Ryan's comfort and confidence increased. His overly assertive and withdrawn behaviors decreased. A successful social functioning Ryan was emerging, and it felt good to Ryan. For Ryan, the combination of the relationship group environment with the opportunity to practice social skills through play interventions gave him what he had been needing and wanting. By the end of the group, Ryan was a fully engaged, social preadolescent that wasn't feeling rejected any longer and had five new friends which he continued to socialize with after the group ended.

AutPlay groups are not just about addressing social skill deficits and implementing structured interventions to improve deficits. This component is certainly present, but this alone does not provide the full description of AutPlay groups. Indeed, the heart of an AutPlay group has more to do with Ryan's journey than any particular social skill intervention. The true definition of success in an AutPlay group is the ability of a childlike Ryan to find hope, confidence, and success with who he is as a social being and success in navigating his social world.

The ability for a childlike Ryan to experience enjoyment in a social world that has historically represented hurt and confusion is the greatest testament to the success of AutPlay groups. It represents the value and importance of facilitating AutPlay groups in communities across the world and providing more narratives like Ryan's experience. The more

Ryan stories that can be written, the more children will heal from social rejection and find a place of peace in their social world. AutPlay play and social skills groups provide the design and protocol for professionals to assist children and adolescents in gaining the skills they need while respecting and valuing them as unique individuals. The ultimate accomplishment of AutPlay groups is helping these children feel confident and secure in social navigation.

Key Terms

Chapter 1

- Autism Spectrum Disorder (ASD): A broad range of conditions characterized by challenges with social skills, repetitive behaviors, speech, and nonverbal communication.
- Individualized Educational Program (IEP): A legal document under United States law that is developed for each public-school child in the U.S. who needs special education.
- 504 Plan: A plan developed to ensure that a child who has a disability identified under the law and is attending an elementary or secondary educational institution receives accommodations.
- DSM V: The Diagnostic and Statistical Manual of Mental Disorders, Fifth Edition. The tool used for diagnosing mental conditions.
- Levels of support: The three levels of support to distinguish Autism Spectrum Disorder.
- Splinter skills: Abilities that are disconnected from their usual context or are very specific abilities that do not generalize to other capabilities.
- Uneven development: Differences in areas of development.
- Receptive language: A person's ability to take in and receive language.
- Generalization: The tendency to respond in the same way across multiple situations and environments.
- Rigid thinking: Literal thinking with concrete thoughts.
- Executive functioning: A set of cognitive processes that are necessary for the cognitive control of behavior.
- Processing speed: The time it takes a person to do a mental task.
- Emotional regulation: The process by which individuals influence which emotions they have, when they have them, and how they experience and express them.
- Perseveration: The act of repeating or "getting stuck" carrying out a behavior, thought, or vocalization when it is no longer appropriate.
- Eye gaze: Looking at the face of others to check and see what they are looking at and to signal interest in interacting.

- Theory of mind: The understanding that others have beliefs, desires, and intentions that are different from one's own, and that is acceptable.
- Joint attention: The shared focus of two individuals on an object.
- Social reciprocity: The back and forth flow of social interaction.
- Introspection: The ability to self-reflect and process on one's thoughts and emotions.
- Self-advocacy: An individual's ability to effectively communicate, convey, negotiate or assert his or her own interests, desires, needs, and rights.

Chapter 2

- Social competence: A complex set of skills that evolves over the course of human development.
- Social skill: A general term referring to a variety of social abilities, from simple to complex.
- Social functioning: The ability to be skilled and successful in social environments.
- Pivotal Response Training: A naturalistic form of applied behavior analysis used as an early intervention for children with autism.
- Social narratives: Also known as social stories, creating a narrative around a child's particular social difficulty.
- Social cognition: How people process, store, and apply information about other people and social situations.
- Receptive language: A person's ability to take in and receive language.
- Social reciprocity: The back and forth interactions that make up all social encounters.
- AutPlay Social Skills Inventory: An inventory developed to help assess a child or adolescent's social skill strengths and deficits.
- Group Readiness Questionnaire: A questionnaire developed to determine a child or adolescent's readiness to participate in AutPlay Therapy groups.

Chapter 3

- Therapeutic factors of play: Also known as the 20 core agents of change from the book: *The Therapeutic Powers of Play: 20 Core Agents of Change, 2nd Edition*
- Expressive communication: The use of words, sentences, gestures, and writing to convey meaning and messages to others.
- Abreaction: A psychoanalytical term for reliving an experience to purge it of its emotional excesses.
- Cognitive development: A child's development in terms of information processing, conceptual resources, perceptual skill, and language learning.

- Social skills: A general term referring to a variety of social abilities, from simple to complex.
- AutPlay Therapy: Developed by Dr. Robert Jason Grant, a therapy approach that involves a combination of behavioral and relational approaches for working with children and adolescents with ASD, developmental disorders, and other neurodevelopmental disorders.
- AutPlay Social Skills Inventory: An inventory developed to help assess a child or adolescent's social skill strengths and deficits.
- AutPlay Therapy Follow Me Approach (FMA): An approach used for clients with lower functioning connection or social skills.

Chapter 4

- AutPlay Group Formation Guide: A guide that helps with the planning of preparing for AutPlay Therapy groups.
- AutPlay Therapy groups: A specific type of skill building groups that can help children and adolescents develop relationships, practice skills, and have positive recreational experiences.
- Therapeutic relationship development: Purposeful positioning and response on the part of the professional that enables the child to feel safe, free to explore, express, and discover what the child needs in order to heal.
- Playful flow: An immersion in play where a children lose their sense of self-awareness and become caught up in the process.
- Structured play: Play that is based on directive activities.
- Dysregulation: The inability to manage the intensity and duration of difficult emotions.
- AutPlay Therapy limit setting model: A limit setting model that follows the three R's Redirect, Replace, and Removal.
- ACT limit setting model: A limit setting model that follows three steps: Acknowledge what the child wants, needs or is feeling; Communicate the limit in a non-punitive manner; and Target acceptable alternatives for the child.
- Filial Therapy limit setting model: A limit setting model that follows three steps: The professional states the limit, gives a warning, and enforces the consequence.
- Adlerian limit setting model: A limit setting model that follows four steps: Stating the limit, reflecting the child's feelings, generating acceptable alternatives, and logical consequences.

Chapter 5

- Follow Me Approach (FMA): An AutPlay Therapy approach used with children who have a functioning level that creates issues with focusing on and being able to participate in directive play therapy interventions as well as children who are too young to participate in directive interventions.

- AutPlay play groups: Groups designed for preschool aged children who have a diagnosis of autism or related condition. They are also appropriate for children of this age who are struggling with social interaction. AutPlay play groups provide an atmosphere of playful interaction facilitated by a professional and includes parent participation.
- Session Overview Form: A form used in AutPlay play groups to summarize the session and give details on practice and location of parent-led sessions.
- Limit setting model: A plan on how to handle unwanted behavior in a group setting.

Chapter 6

- AutPlay social skills groups: Social skills groups based off the directive phase of AutPlay Therapy. These groups focus on improving social functioning and are designed for elementary, middle, and high school aged children who have been diagnosed with autism or a related condition.
- Session Overview Form: A form used in AutPlay play groups to summarize the session and give details on practice and location of parent-led sessions.
- Limit setting model: A plan on how to handle unwanted behavior in a group setting.
- Co-change agents: In the chapter, a term used to describe the parents. Their participation in groups helps the children transform in their social skill development.

Chapter 7

- AutPlay social skills groups: Social skills groups based off the directive phase of AutPlay Therapy. These groups focus on improving social functioning and are designed for elementary, middle, and high school aged children who have been diagnosed with autism or a related condition.
- Social skills: A general term referring to a variety of social abilities, from simple to complex.
- Social skills activity: An intervention using play designed to help improve social skill functioning in children and/or adolescents.

Appendix
Step-by-Step Guide for Implementing AutPlay Groups

1. Group Structure—Establish a group meeting location, any support professional that will be working with you to facilitate the group, and what your group fee will be. These components can vary greatly and should be decided on by the professional depending on his or her work setting.
2. Market Your Group—Establish the age range and/or functioning level of the group members, establish this before marketing a group and target the type of group being offered. Also, decide and indicate on marketing materials if it will be a play group or a social skills group or possibly both. Otherwise began a general marketing effort and see who signs up and form the group(s) accordingly.
3. Meet with the Parents and Child—As people indicate an interest in participating in a group, meet with the parent and child. This is a time to get more information about the child and observe the child. The parent should complete the Intake Form, Group Readiness Form, Confidentiality Form, Social Skills Inventory, and any additional paperwork that is needed. After this meeting and upon review of the completed forms, the professional should make one of the following decisions regarding participation in a group:

   • Sign the child up for a group that is beginning.
   • Place the child on a waiting list for when an appropriate group begins.
   • Discuss with the parent that the child is not ready for a group and offer individual therapy or a referral.

4. Establish the Schedule—Once the group members have been selected, complete the group schedule. Establish with the parents who will be hosting a meeting outside of the clinic and when this will take place—make sure to indicate these dates on the Group Schedule Form. The parents should be given the completed Group Schedule Form before the first group meeting. This schedule will show parents when in clinic groups are happening and when a parent hosting meeting is happening. Also, give parents the Participants Contact Information

Form. This will enable parents to contact other parents when hosting an outside of the clinic meeting.

5. First Session—Begin the first group session in the clinic location. Follow the group meetings guide in this book. Remember this is just a guide, the professional has the flexibility to add, integrate, and adapt from the guide. Once group sessions begin, it is a consistent and organized routine that happens week to week until the 20 meetings have ended.

6. Session Overview Form—At the end of each session, the professional should give the parents the Session Overview Form. This form highlights what was worked on in the session, how to continue to support social skill development at home, and information about the next weeks parent hosted meeting. The professional should have the form completed before the group begins for easy distribution to all the parents at the end of the group meeting.

7. Continue with groups two through ten following the group meetings guide in this book. Again, remember this is a guide and the professional may adapt or integrate protocol throughout the 10 meetings. This is something the professional will decide based on what they feel is appropriate and helpful for their groups. AutPlay Groups have an intentional looseness to give professionals the ability to individualize their groups based on their expertise and the needs of the children and adolescents in the group.

8. Group 10 will be the last group meeting and should provide closure for the group. The group meeting guide in this book provides information on terminating the group. Professionals should consider if it would be beneficial for a group to continue to meet. In some cases, 10 meetings will not be enough for a child or adolescent to achieve their social skill goals. The professional could decide to continue the group for an additional set amount of sessions, continue the group indefinitely, start another group with some previous group participants and some new participants. Often with AutPlay Play Groups, because of the severity of impairment the children possess, these groups could easily continue beyond the ten meetings and be of benefit to the children.

AutPlay Groups Sample Marketing Letter

Date:

Dear Parent/Guardian of _____:

Hello. My name is _____, and I am beginning an AutPlay Social Skills group. AutPlay Therapy is a behavioral play therapy approach to working with children and adolescents with autism spectrum disorder and other developmental disabilities. AutPlay Therapy focuses on improving a child's emotional regulation, social skills development, and relationship development and connection. It has also been shown to reduce anxiety, improve sensory processing challenges, increase concentration, focus and attention, reduce unwanted behaviors and improve the parent/child relationship. An AutPlay Social Skills group will work specifically on social skills activities that will help the group members improve their interactions with other peers.

This group will meet weekly on _____ at _____. In addition to in-clinic sessions, there will also be weekly groups hosted by each parent. This is a fun and informative way for the group members to further practice their skills, while parents have the opportunity to get to know each other and learn more about how to facilitate social skills activities. There will also be ideas given to parents on how to practice essential social skills at home.

Please complete the form below if you are interested in your child attending this group. I will need the form returned to me by _____.

Thank you for your interest!

Sincerely,

_____cut here_____

I give permission for my child, _____, to attend the AutPlay Therapy Social Skills Group. I understand this group meets in-clinic weekly and will also have parent-hosted groups. I am willing to host one of these groups.

_____   _____
Parent Signature   Date

Contact us at _____

_____

AutPlay Groups Intake Form Page One

Name: _____ Date of Birth: _____

Parent(s)/Guardian(s) Name(s):_____

Address: _____
        Street number and name   City   State   Zip Code

Phone Number: (___)_____ Okay to leave a message? Yes or No (circle one)

Email Address: _____

In Case of Emergency Notify: _____ Phone: (___)_____

Primary Care Physician: _____ Phone: (___)_____

List any and all diagnosis your child has received:_____
_____

List any medical problems that I need to be aware of: _____
_____

List all medications that are currently being prescribed: _____
_____

List any allergies, including food allergies/sensitivities: _____
_____

Does your child have any sensory processing challenges:_____
_____

Describe your child's social skills difficulties: _____
_____
_____
_____
_____

Describe your child's social skills strengths: _____
_____
_____
_____
_____

AutPlay Groups Intake Form Page Two

Fee and Payment Information

Fees for group sessions are due and payable on the day of service unless other arrangements are made prior to the time of service. Cash, credit card, and checks are accepted. Many insurance plans are accepted. Clients should consult their insurance provider for information regarding co-payment, deductible, and number of authorized sessions. Regardless of what an insurance company states to this office or you about payment for services, this is not a guarantee of payment for services. You are still responsible for full payment for group services even if an insurance company states they will pay and do not.

Co-pays must be paid at the time of the session. If the office must mail you an invoice, then a processing fee of $_____ will be applied. Co-pays can be paid to the front office staff or your therapist. A copy of your insurance card should be on file with this office.

Medicaid and MC+ are accepted. A copy of the Medicaid or MC+ card should be on file with this office. The average group session time lasts one hour. The standard fee per group session is $_____.

Medicaid

Name of Child on Medicaid Card:_____

Medicaid Number:_____ Birth Date:_____

Private Insurance

Name of Responsible Party on Insurance Card:_____

Parent Social Security #_____Child Social Security #_____

Insurance Company/Plan:_____

Individual #_____ Group #_____

Insurance Company Billing Address & Phone Number: _____

_____

_____

_____

I have read and understood the above related fee payment information and agree to the terms defined by this office.

_____

Client Name	Guardian/Client Signature	Date

AutPlay Groups Intake Form Page Three

Cancelation of Sessions and No-Show Sessions

If a group meeting is scheduled and needs to be canceled, you must cancel by phone prior to the scheduled group meeting time. If you fail to cancel before the scheduled group meeting time, you will be charged a $_____ fee that must be paid before continuing with sessions. Further, if a group meeting is missed with no cancelation made, you are not guaranteed a continued spot in the group. It is your responsibility to contact this office if a group meeting needs to be canceled and to verify any future group meetings. Exceptions to these guidelines include a crisis situation, emergency, disaster, or unexpected illness.

Record Requests and Release

Minimal records are kept regarding group meetings, but basic intake, consent, and session notes are maintained. You may ask to see your child's records or request a copy of your child's records at any time. We do require a seven-day notice for a records request. You may also request a report be written to a third party at any time. Requests for a report of any type must be given at least seven days in advance. We cannot guarantee any request for a report that has been submitted with less than a seven-day notice—the report will likely not be provided by the requested date. Please note that when requesting a specific report be written, a reasonable fee will be charged for providing a copy of your report or a summary of records which would include cost of copying, postage, and preparation or an explanation or summary of the information.

Court-Related Records, Testimony, and Appearance

If the therapist is requested or subpoenaed at any point in time to appear in court or participate in court-related activities on you or your child's behalf, you will be responsible for payment reimbursement of the therapist's time which will be billed at a rate of $_____ per hour. Travel time spent to and from court or other venues related to court activities will be considered part of the hourly time billed. If records or documents are requested or subpoenaed, a reasonable fee will be charged for providing a copy of your records or a summary of those records which would include cost of copying, postage, and preparation or an explanation or summary of the information.

I have read and understood the above related fee payment information and court related information and agree to the terms defined by this office.

_____   _____   _____
Client Name   Guardian/Client Signature   Date

AutPlay Groups Confidentiality Statement

All persons participating in group counseling must read and sign this agreement. If you do not understand any part of this agreement, please ask any questions prior to signing the agreement.

Confidentiality

Anything said between group members at any time is part of the group and is confidential. I understand that everything said in this group is confidential and not to be shared with anyone outside of the group, except as may be otherwise required by law. I understand this includes in clinic group meetings as well as parent-hosted outside clinic group meetings and play times.

- I agree to keep confidential the names of other members of the group and what is said in the group. As a member of this group, I agree to not disclose to anyone outside the group any information that may identify another group member. This includes, but is not limited to, names, physical descriptions, biological information, and specifics to the content of interactions with other group members.
- I agree to indemnify and hold _____ harmless for any loss or damages, including costs and attorney's fees, incurred by _____ as a result of my breach of another's confidentiality.

I also understand that anything said in group therapy is confidential, *except* for the following limitations:

- Child abuse and/or neglect.
- Vulnerable adult abuse or neglect.
- Threats to harm oneself.
- Threats regarding harm to another person.
- A court subpoena.
- My specific request, in writing, to disclose information regarding my psychotherapy to a third party.

Please note that if you choose to send communications through text or email these communications are not protected and confidentiality cannot be assured.

By my signature below, I indicate that I have read carefully and understand the AutPlay Group Therapy Confidentiality Statement and I agree to its terms and conditions. I am aware signing the Agreement is required for my admission to the group. I am also aware that my refusal to sign this Agreement will exclude me from participating in the group.

Guardian/Client Name (print): _____

Guardian/Client Signature: _____

Date:_____

AutPlay Group Readiness Questionnaire Page One

Child Name: _____ Age:_____

Parent(s) Name:_____ Phone:_____

What ASD diagnosis or other diagnosis (if any) does your child have?

Rate your child's social functioning ability on a scale from one to ten, one being extremely low and ten being very high.

Does your child have any physical disabilities or physical needs?

Rate your child's verbal communication ability on a scale from one to ten, one being extremely low and ten being very high.

Has your child ever participated in a social group before? If so, what was the experience like for your child?

What does your child like to do for fun?

What community/public activities has your child participated in that he/she seemed to enjoy?

What are some of your child's interests?

What community/public activities has your child participated in that he/she seemed to not enjoy?

AutPlay Group Readiness Questionnaire Page Two

Child Name:_____ Age:_____

Parent(s) Name:_____ Phone:_____

What sensory issues does your child seem to respond negatively to (large crowds, noise, etc.)?

What social skills would you like to see your child gain or improve?

What do you feel would be your child's biggest challenge in being in a peer social group?

Would your child do well with older children, younger children, children of the opposite gender?

How would you like a social group for your child to assist you as a parent?

Are you willing to participate in the group experience with your child?

Any additional information you would like to share with us about your child?

AutPlay Groups Participants Contact Information

Child's Name _____

Parent's Name and Contact Information _____

_____

Child's Name _____

Parent's Name and Contact Information _____

_____

Child's Name _____

Parent's Name and Contact Information _____

_____

Child's Name _____

Parent's Name and Contact Information _____

_____

Child's Name _____

Parent's Name and Contact Information _____

_____

Child's Name _____

Parent's Name and Contact Information _____

_____

Child's Name _____

Parent's Name and Contact Information _____

_____

Child's Name _____

Parent's Name and Contact Information _____

_____

Child's Name _____

Parent's Name and Contact Information _____

_____

Social Skills Group Schedule				
	CLINIC OR PARENT HOSTED (CIRCLE ONE)	DATE	TIME	ADDITIONAL INFORMATION
Week One	CLINIC PARENT			
Week Two	CLINIC PARENT			
Week Three	CLINIC PARENT			
Week Four	CLINIC PARENT			
Week Five	CLINIC PARENT			
Week Six	CLINIC PARENT			
Week Seven	CLINIC PARENT			
Week Eight	CLINIC PARENT			
Week Nine	CLINIC PARENT			
Week Ten	CLINIC PARENT			
Week Eleven	CLINIC PARENT			
Week Twelve	CLINIC PARENT			
Week Thirteen	CLINIC PARENT			
Week Fourteen	CLINIC PARENT			
Week Fifteen	CLINIC PARENT			
Week Sixteen	CLINIC PARENT			
Week Seventeen	CLINIC PARENT			
Week Eighteen	CLINIC PARENT			
Week Nineteen	CLINIC PARENT			
Week Twenty	CLINIC PARENT			

AutPlay Group Session Overview Form

Date: _____

Group Session Number: _____

Session Summary:_____

Home Practice:_____

Additional Information:_____

Next In-Clinic Session:_____

Next Parent-Hosted Session: _____
  • Name of parent_____
  • Location of event_____

AutPlay Group Session Overview Form—Example

Date: January 25, 2020

Group Session Number: 4

Session Summary: Today's focus was on personal space. We learned how all of us feel comfortable with a different amount of space! It's important to be aware of this, and to ask others if we are giving them enough personal space. We can also look for cues that someone is uncomfortable with how close we are to them (they are backing away from us for example).

Home Practice: Practice personal space in a variety of settings. This can be in a line, having a conversation, going down a slide, etc. You can use a prop, such as a piece of string or a pool noodle to discover how much personal space each family member needs. You can also come up with a special word when you feel you need more space (a word as simple as "Space") and practice using this word as a family.

Additional Information: Personal space can be a difficult concept, so practice it often. Once learned, repeated practice may be needed in a variety of other sessions.

Next In-Clinic Session: February 8, 2020 at 10:00am

Next Parent-Hosted Session: February 1, 2020 at 10:00am

- Name of parent: Janice Jackson
- Location of event: Hubert Park, 123 Main Street

AutPlay Groups Parent Update Form

Please complete this form and provide information about your child's experience and participation in outside of the clinic parent hosted meetings.

Parent's Name: _____

Child's Name: _____

_____

Describe the activity in which your child participated:

_____

Describe any observations about your child's participation:

_____

Describe any challenges or issues you noticed:

_____

Describe any strengths, skill gains, or positives you noticed:

AutPlay Groups Session Note

Child's Name: _____ Date: _____

Group Meeting #: _____ Time: _____ Group Procedure Code: _____

Child' Diagnosis: _____ Group Facilitator: _____

Group members present: _____

_____

_____

_____

Group intervention, approach, or activity (as related to treatment goals):

_____

Child's response to group participation:

_____

Child's progress in group (as related to treatment goals):

_____

Additional information:

_____   _____
Signature of Professional   Date

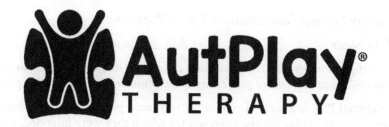

AutPlay® Group Certificate of Completion

This completion certificate is awarded to

Child Name

_____

Parent Name

_____

For successfully completing the AutPlay Therapy Group experience.

Signature of Facilitator   Date

_____   _____

AutPlay Groups Assessment of Play—Page One

Child Name_____Age____Gender____Date_____

Read the following play categories and definitions and rate where you feel your child is at in terms of possessing and demonstrating this type of play.

Functional Play is a term also used for relational play, it means denoting use of objects in play for the purposes for which they were intended, e.g., using simple objects correctly, combining related objects (a female doll in a beauty parlor), and making objects do what they are made to do.
Lacking 1   2   3   4   5   6   7   8   9   10 Demonstrates

Symbolic Play refers to symbolic, or dramatic, play which occurs when children begin to substitute one object for another. For example, using a hairbrush to represent a microphone. The child may pretend to do something (with or without the object present or with an object representing another object) or be someone. They may also pretend through other inanimate objects (e.g., has a doll pretend to feed another doll).
Lacking 1   2   3   4   5   6   7   8   9   10 Demonstrates

Cooperative Play refers to a play where children plan, assign roles and play together. Cooperative play is goal-oriented and children play in an organized manner toward a common end. Moreover, Cooperative play is a "true Social play" in which children cooperate or assume reciprocal roles.
Lacking 1   2   3   4   5   6   7   8   9   10 Demonstrates

Sociodramatic Play refers to play involving acting out scripts, scenes, and plays adopted from cartoons and books. Children take/assume roles using themselves and/or characters like dolls, figures, and puppets as they interact together on common themes. As a child matures, themes, sequences, plans, problem solving, characters and so forth become richer and they begin to organize other children for role play with independence.
Lacking 1   2   3   4   5   6   7   8   9   10 Demonstrates

Peer play refers to interactions with one's peers, which provide opportunities for physical, cognitive, social, and emotional development.
Lacking 1   2   3   4   5   6   7   8   9   10 Demonstrates

Constructive Play characterized as manipulation of objects for the purpose of constructing or creating something. Children use materials to achieve a specific goal in mind that requires transformation of objects into a new configuration. Lego pieces turned to cars or houses are an example of this play.
Lacking 1   2   3   4   5   6   7   8   9   10 Demonstrates

Representational Play refers to pretend play which emerges when a child begins to use familiar objects in appropriate ways to represent their world, an example is a cooking gas toy where a food is being cooked.
Lacking 1   2   3   4   5   6   7   8   9   10 Demonstrates

Child Name_____ Age_____ Gender_____ Date_____

Please answer the following questions regarding your child's play. Try to think about specific times you have observed or played with your child and answer the questions as completely as possible.

Does your child play with toys?

Does your child play independently?

Does your child play with other children?

Does your child initiate play with other children or adults?

Do you have play times with your child?

Does your child interact with you during play times?

Does your child do pretend play or metaphor play?

Does your child play with objects that would not be considered toys?

If someone (child or adult) asks your child to play, what does your child usually do?

Does your child seem to want to play?

Does your child's play seem age appropriate?

Describe your child's play.

Play categories in part from Psychology Glossary (2012), www.psychology-lexicon.com

AutPlay Groups Social Skills Inventory—Child (3–11)

Name _____ Age____ Gender ____ Date _____

Rate the following social skills on the continuum from not developed to developed, with 1 being not developed at all and 5 being sufficiently developed.

SKILL	Not Developed			Developed	
Says hello to others	1	2	3	4	5
Makes eye contact with others	1	2	3	4	5
Plays with other children	1	2	3	4	5
Shows kindness to others	1	2	3	4	5
Shares with others	1	2	3	4	5
Listens without interrupting	1	2	3	4	5
Asks questions	1	2	3	4	5
Answers questions when asked	1	2	3	4	5
Talks about feelings	1	2	3	4	5
Shows appropriate body language	1	2	3	4	5
Understands other people's body language	1	2	3	4	5
Asks for help	1	2	3	4	5
Follows rules	1	2	3	4	5
Includes other children in his or her play	1	2	3	4	5
Understands other's point of view	1	2	3	4	5
Handles anger/frustration	1	2	3	4	5
Asks to play with other children	1	2	3	4	5
Understands teasing and bullying	1	2	3	4	5
Ignores teasing and bullying	1	2	3	4	5
Speaks in appropriate tone of voice	1	2	3	4	5
Speaks at appropriate rate	1	2	3	4	5
Speaks clearly	1	2	3	4	5
Feels sorry for inappropriate behaviors	1	2	3	4	5
Responds when spoken to	1	2	3	4	5
Understands social boundaries	1	2	3	4	5
Knows safety information	1	2	3	4	5
Has friends his or her own age	1	2	3	4	5
Knows how to make friends	1	2	3	4	5
Asks other children to play with him or her	1	2	3	4	5
Accepts response of "no"	1	2	3	4	5
Ignores distractions	1	2	3	4	5
Understands appropriate behaviors in public	1	2	3	4	5
Expresses a desire to play with peers	1	2	3	4	5
Talks appropriately (not too much or too little)	1	2	3	4	5
Understands manner	1	2	3	4	5

SKILL	Not Developed			Developed	
Participates appropriately in peer groups	1	2	3	4	5
Talks to adults	1	2	3	4	5
Acknowledges other people's presence	1	2	3	4	5
Solves problems	1	2	3	4	5
Verbally expresses feelings	1	2	3	4	5

AutPlay Groups Social Skills Inventory—Adolescent (12–18)

Name_____ Age____ Gender ____ Date_____

Rate the following social skills on the continuum from not developed to developed, with 1 being not developed at all and 5 being sufficiently developed.

SKILL	Not Developed			Developed	
Introduces self to others	1	2	3	4	5
Makes eye contact with others	1	2	3	4	5
Socializes with other children his or her age	1	2	3	4	5
Shows empathy to others	1	2	3	4	5
Shares with others	1	2	3	4	5
Listens without interrupting	1	2	3	4	5
Identifies needs in others and will help	1	2	3	4	5
Asks for help	1	2	3	4	5
Talks about feelings	1	2	3	4	5
Displays appropriate body language	1	2	3	4	5
Understands other's body language	1	2	3	4	5
Ends a conversation	1	2	3	4	5
Enters a conversation	1	2	3	4	5
Includes others in what he or she is doing	1	2	3	4	5
Understands other's point of view	1	2	3	4	5
Handles anger/frustration appropriately	1	2	3	4	5
Knows how to join a group	1	2	3	4	5
Follows rules	1	2	3	4	5
Knows how to compromise	1	2	3	4	5
Speaks in appropriate tone of voice	1	2	3	4	5
Speaks at appropriate rate	1	2	3	4	5
Accepts response of no	1	2	3	4	5
Accepts responsibility for actions	1	2	3	4	5
Responds when spoken to	1	2	3	4	5
Knows appropriate social boundaries	1	2	3	4	5
Knows safety information	1	2	3	4	5
Expresses own opinions	1	2	3	4	5
Makes friends with others	1	2	3	4	5
Can initiate tasks on own	1	2	3	4	5
Expresses concern for others	1	2	3	4	5
Ignores distractions	1	2	3	4	5
Can give directions	1	2	3	4	5
Can explain things to others	1	2	3	4	5
Apologizes for mistakes	1	2	3	4	5
Understands manners	1	2	3	4	5
Cooperates and participates in peer groups	1	2	3	4	5
Talks to adults	1	2	3	4	5
Understands teasing and bullying	1	2	3	4	5

SKILL	Not Developed			Developed	
Solves problems	1	2	3	4	5
Uses appropriate hygiene	1	2	3	4	5

Feelings List

Accepted	Afraid	Affectionate	Loyal
Angry	Miserable	Anxious	Misunderstood
Peaceful	Beautiful	Playful	Ashamed
Brave	Awkward	Calm	Proud
Capable	Quite	Bored	Overwhelmed
Caring	Relaxed	Confused	Cheerful
Relieved	Defeated	Comfortable	Safe
Competent	Satisfied	Concerned	Mad
Depressed	Pressured	Confident	Provoked
Content	Desperate	Regretful	Courageous
Silly	Lonely	Rejected	Curious
Special	Disappointed	Remorseful	Strong
Discouraged	Disgusted	Sad	Sympathetic
Excited	Embarrassed	Shy	Forgiving
Thankful	Sorry	Friendly	Thrilled
Fearful	Stubborn	Nervous	Stupid
Glad	Understood	Frustrated	Good
Unique	Furious	Tired	Grateful
Valuable	Guilty	Touchy	Great
Hateful	Happy	Helpless	Hopeful
Wonderful	Hopeless	Humorous	Worthwhile
Unattractive	Joyful	Uncertain	Lovable
Humiliated	Uncomfortable	Loved	Hurt
Ignored	Impatient	Indecisive	Inferior
Insecure	Irritated	Jealous	Worried

Social Skills List

- Listening
- Starting a Conversation
- Ending a Conversation
- Introducing Self
- Introducing Other People
- Asking For Help
- Apologizing
- Sharing
- Helping Others
- Appropriate Body Language
- Understanding Personal Space
- Making and Maintaining Friends
- Handling Losing
- Giving Instructions
- Negotiating
- Handling Bullying
- Accepting Consequences
- Recognizing Trouble Situations
- Completing Tasks Without Assistance
- Well-Rounded Play Skills
- Flexibility
- Expressing Emotions Appropriately
- Recognizing Emotions in Others
- Expressing Concern for Others
- Emotion/Situation Appropriateness
- Handling Anger Related Feelings
- Dealing with Accusation
- Self-Relaxation Techniques
- Other_____

- Asking Questions
- Smiling
- Saying Thank You
- Making Eye Contact
- Basic Boundaries
- Following Instructions
- Asking Permission
- Joining in a Group
- Taking Turns
- Appropriate Tone of Voice
- Two-Way Conversation
- Public Boundaries
- Handling Winning
- Convincing Others
- Using Self Control
- Giving Compliments
- ManagingDisagreements
- Understanding Humor
- Initiating Tasks
- Problem Solving
- Advanced Boundaries
- Knowing Emotions
- Expressing Affection
- Handling Anxiety
- Showing Compassion
- Avoiding Fights
- Standing Up for Others
- Accepting "No"

_____
_____

Additional Group Resources

Ashcroft, W., Delloso, A. M., & Quinn, A. M. (2013). *Social skills games & activities for kids with autism*. Prufrock Press.

Denning, C. (2017). *Developing motor and social skills: Activities for children with autism spectrum disorder*. Rowman & Littlefield.

Grant, R. J. (2017). *AutPlay Therapy for children and adolescents on the autism spectrum: A behavioral play-based approach*. (3rd ed.). Routledge.

Grant, R. J. (2017). *Play-based interventions for autism spectrum disorders*. Routledge.

Hull K. B. (2014). *Group therapy techniques with children, adolescents, and adults on the autism spectrum: Growth and connection for all ages*. Jason Aronson.

Hull, K. B. (2011). *Play therapy and Asperger's syndrome: Helping children and adolescents grow, connect, and heal through the art of play*. Jason Aronson.

Koenig, K. (2012). *Practical social skills for autism spectrum disorders*. W. W. Norton.

LeGoff, D. B., De La Cuesta, G. G., Krauss, G. W., & Baron-Cohen, S. (2014). *LEGO®-based therapy*. Jessica Kingsley Publishers.

Pascuas, C. (2017). *Social skills handbook for autism: Activities to help kids learn social skills and make friends*. Autism Handbooks.

Simpson, R. L., & McGinnis-Smith, E. (2018). *Social skills success for students with Asperger syndrome and high-functioning autism*. Corwin.

Sweeney, D. S., Baggerly, J. N., & Ray, D. C. (2014). *Group play therapy: A dynamic approach*. Routledge.

Sweeney, D. S., & Homeyer, L. (1999). *Handbook of group play therapy: How to do it, how it works, whom it's best for*. Jossey-Bass.

References

American Psychological Association. (2014). *Diagnostic and statistical manual of mental disorders (5th ed.)*. Author.

Ashcroft, W., Delloso, A. M., & Quinn, A. M. (2013). *Social skills games & activities for kids with autism*. Prufrock Press.

Association for Play Therapy. (2019). *Play therapy best practices*. www.a4pt.org/page/Publications.

Attwood, T., & Garnett, M. (2013). *CBT to help young people with Asperger's syndrome (autism spectrum disorder) to understand and express affection*. Jessica Kingsley Publishers.

Autism Society of America (2020). Wh*at is autism*. www.autism-society.org/.

Barboa, L. & Luck, J. (2016). *The nuts and bolts of autism: Just the facts*. KIP Publishing.

Booth, P. B., & Jernberg, A. M. (2010). *Theraplay*. Jossey-Bass.

Centers for Disease Control and Prevention (2020). *What is autism spectrum disorder*. www.cdc.gov/ncbddd/autism/index.html.

Coplan, J. (2010). *Making sense of autistic spectrum disorders*. Bantam Books.

Cross, A. (2010). *Come and play: sensory integration strategies for children with play challenges*. Redleaf Press.

Dawson, G., McPartland, J., & Ozonoff, S. (2002). *A parent's guide to Asperger's syndrome & high functioning autism*. The Guilford Press.

D'Amico, M., & Lalonde, C. (2017). The effectiveness of art therapy for teaching social skills to children with autism spectrum disorder. *Art Therapy: Journal of the American Art Therapy Association*, 34(4) pp. 176–182.

Dienstmann, R. (2008). *Games for motor learning*. Champaign, IL: Human Kinetics.

Grandin, T. (2008). *The way I see it: A personal look at autism and Asperger's*. Future Horizons.

Grant, R. J. (2017). *AutPlay Therapy for children and adolescents on the autism spectrum*. (3rd ed.). Routledge.

Grant, R. J. (2017). *Play-based interventions for Autism spectrum disorders*. Routledge.

Grant, R. J. (2018). *Understanding autism spectrum disorder: a workbook for children and teens*. AutPlay Publishing.

Grant, R. J. (2019). Play therapy for children with autism spectrum disorder. In H. Kaduson, D. Cangelosi, and C. Schaefer (Eds.) *Prescriptive play therapy: Tailoring interventions for specific childhood problems*, pp. 213–230. The Guilford Press.

Greenspan, S., & Wieder, S. (2006). *Engaging autism.* Da Capo Press.

Higashida, N. (2013). *The reason I jump: The inner voice of a thirteen-year-old boy with autism.* Random House.

Jamison, T. R., & Schuttler. J. O. (2017). Overview and preliminary evidence for a social skills and self-care curriculum for adolescent females with autism: The girls night out model. *Journal of Autism Developmental Disorders,* 47, pp. 110–125.

Kasari, C., Dean, M., Kretzmann, M., Shih, W., Orlich, F., Whitney, R., Landa, R., Lord, C., & King, B. (2016). Children with autism spectrum disorder and social skills groups at school: a randomized trial comparing intervention approach and peer composition. *Journal of Child Psychology and Psychiatry,* 57(2) pp. 171–179.

Knell. S. M. (1997). *Cognitive behavioral play therapy.* Rowman and Littlefield.

Koenig, K. (2012). *Practical social skills for autism spectrum disorders.* W. W. Norton.

Kottman, T. (2011). *Play therapy: Basics and beyond.* American Counseling Association.

Kottman, T. (2003). *Partners in Play: An Adlerian Approach to Play Therapy.* American Counseling Association.

Landreth, G. L. (1991). *Play therapy: The art of the relationship.* Brunner-Routledge.

Lara, J. (2016). *Autism movement therapy method: Waking up the brain.* Jessica Kingsley Publishers.

Leaf, J. B., Leaf, J. A., Milne, C., Taubman, M., Oppenheim-Leaf, M., Torres, N., Townley-Cochran, D., Leaf, R., John McEachin, J., & Yoder, P. (2017). An evaluation of a behaviorally based social skills group for individuals diagnosed with autism spectrum disorder. *Journal of Autism Developmental Disorders,* 47, pp. 243–259.

LeGoff, D. B., De La Cuesta, G. G., Krauss, G. W., & Baron-Cohen, S. (2014). *LEGO®-based therapy.* Jessica Kingsley Publishers.

Levine, K., & Chedd, N. (2006). *Replays: Using play to enhance emotional and behavioral development for children with autism spectrum disorders.* Jessica Kingsley Publishers.

MacDonald, J. & Stoika P. (2007). *Play to talk: A practical guide to help your late-talking child join the conversation.* Kiddo Publishing.

McCloud, C. (2015). *Have you filled a bucket today: A guide to daily happiness for kids.* Bucket Filler Publishing.

Mellenthin, C. (2018). *Play therapy: Engaging & powerful techniques for the treatment of childhood disorders.* PESI Publishing.

Milestones Autism Resources. (2020). *What is autism.* www.milestones.org/.

Murphy, A. N., Radley, K. C., & Helbig, K. A. (2018). Use of superheroes social skills with middle school-age students with autism spectrum disorder. *Psychology in the Schools.* 55:323–335.

Murphy. M., Burns, J., & Kilbey, E. (2017). Using personal construct methodology to explore relationships with adolescents with autism spectrum disorder. *Research in Developmental Disabilities,* 70, pp. 22–32.

Phillips, N. & Beavan, L. (2010). *Teaching play to children with autism.* Sage Publications.

Prizant, B. M., Wetherby, A. M., Rubin, E., Laurent, A. C., & Rydell, P. J. (2006). *The SCERTS model: A comprehensive educational approach for children with autism spectrum disorders*. Paul H Brookes Publishing.

Radley, K. C., Hanglein, J., & Arak, M. (2016). School-based social skills training for school age children with autism spectrum disorder. *Autism*, 20, pp. 938–951.

Reichow, B., & Volkmar, F. R. (2010). Social skills interventions for individuals with autism: Evaluation for evidence-based practices within a best evidence synthesis framework. *Journal of Autism and Developmental Disorders*, 40, 149–166.

Schaefer, C. E. & Drewes, A. A. (2014). *The therapeutic powers of play: 20 core agents of change*. Wiley and Sons.

Schaefer, C.E. (2003). *Foundations of play therapy*. John Wiley and Sons Inc.

Siri, K., & Lyons, T. (2010). *Cutting edge therapies for autism*. Skyhorse Publishing.

Stewart, A. L., & Echterling, L. G. (2014). Play and the therapeutic relationship. In C. Schaefer and A. Drewes (Eds.) *The therapeutic powers of play* (2nd ed.), pp. 157–169. Wiley & Sons.

Sweeney, D. S., Baggerly, J. N., & Ray, D. C. (2014). *Group play therapy: A dynamic approach*. Routledge.

Syriopoulou-Delli, C. K., Agaliotis, I., & Papaefstathiou, E. (2018). Social skills characteristics of students with autism spectrum disorder. *International Journal of Developmental Disabilities*. 64(1).

Turner-Bumberry, T. (2019). *2,4,6,8 this is how we regulate: 75 play therapy activities to increase mindfulness in children*. PESI Publishing.

VanFleet, R. (2014). *Filial Therapy: strengthening parent-child relationships through play*. (3rd Ed.). Professional Resource Press.

Ware, J. N., Ohrt, J. H., & Swank, J. M. (2012). A phenomenological exploration of children's experiences in a social skills group. *The Journal for Specialists in Group Work*, 37(2), 133–151.

Wolfberg, P. (2016). Integrated play groups model: Supporting children with autism in essential play experiences with typical peers. In L. A. Reddy, T. M. Files-Hall, & C. E. Schaefer (Eds.), *Empirically based play interventions for children* pp. 223–240. American Psychological Association.

Index

Note: Page numbers in **bold** indicate a table on the corresponding page.

10-session guide: for in clinic AutPlay play groups 50–69; for in clinic AutPlay social skills groups 76–129
504 plan 7

Act As If activity, for adolescents 177
ACT limit setting model, in Child Centered Play Therapy 36–37
Adlerian play therapist, components of 30, 38
adolescents with autism *see* children and adolescents with ASD; interventions (social skills), for adolescents
Agaliotis, I. 16
Animal Charades game 99
Animal Feelings activity, for children 155–156
Animal Pairs activity, for children 136–137
anxiety 16–17, 19; handling 177; reduction 26; struggle with 13
Architects activity, for adolescents 188–189
Ashcroft, W. 17
Association of Play Therapy (APT) 41
Autism Society of America 5
autism spectrum disorder (ASD) 1, 5–15; approaches/procedure to working with 3, 7, 14; behaviors associated with 5; as developmental disability 5; diagnosis of 5–6, 7–9; DSM 5 diagnosis 7–9; social difficulties 18; struggle areas 10–13; symptom of 16; *see also* children and adolescents with ASD
AutPlay® Therapy: ACT limit setting model in 36–37; directive play

therapy interventions 70; ethical considerations for group processes 40–42; Follow Me Approach (FMA) 27–28, 43–44, **44**, 49, 54; formal assessment process in 14; groups, types 3–4, 27, 28, 29–42; interventions 31, 70; limit setting models 35–38; parent training component 26–27; protocol 23, 25–27; for social functioning 26, 31; and social skills 22–28; for working with children with ASD 25; *see also* AutPlay® Therapy play groups; AutPlay® Therapy social skills groups
AutPlay® Therapy play groups 3–4, 28, 29–42, 43–69; 10-session model 50–69; assessing group members 45–46; definition of 45; generating interest in group 45; group meetings 46–47, **48**; group size 46; handling unwanted behavior 48–49; meeting places for parent-hosted groups 47–48, **48**; organization of group 45; parents as co-change agents 49; participation 46; play development 47; pragmatics of 45–49; for preschool-aged/older children 44–45, 46; role of professional 45; social skill development 47; structure 45
AutPlay® Therapy social skills groups 3–4, 17–18, 21, 22–28, 29–42, 32–33, 70–129; 10-session model 76–129; assessing group members 71–72; definition of 71; developing social skills 73; directive interventions phase 70; generating

interest in group 71; group meetings 72–73; group size 72; handling unwanted behavior 74–75; meeting places for parent-hosted groups 73–74, **74**; organization of group 71; parents as co-change agents 75; participation 72; play development 73; pragmatics of 71–75; role of professional 71; structure 71; *see also* interventions (social skills), for adolescents; interventions (social skills), for children
AutPlay Group Formation Guide 29, 30
AutPlay Groups Assessment of Play Form 47, 73
AutPlay Social Skills Inventory 21, 26

Backward Moves activity, for children 165–166
Barboa, L. 18
Bingo Friends activity, for children 138–139
Boatman activity, for children 147–148
"Bring Back My Bonny" song 114
Bubbles Social Skills activity, for children 140–141
Bubble Tag activity, for adolescents 167–168

Centers for Disease Control and Prevention 5
Child Centered Play Therapy 23, 36–37
children and adolescents with ASD 1–2; academic and school related challenges to 6–7; AutPlay interventions at home 26–27; benefits for implementing social skills groups for 70; communication struggles 18–19; deficits in developing relationships 7–8; deficits in social communication and social interaction 7; deficits in social skills 17; dysregulation issues 33–35; expecting from 13–14; implementing social skills intervention 2–3; learning skills through change agents 26; participating in AutPlay groups 21, 29–30, 46, 72; in peer groups 17, 23, 198; play as learning tool for 22; risk for rejection and victimization in school 17; on social

skill improvement 17; social skills intervention for 2–3, 4, 32–33, 38, 77; struggle areas 10–13
Circle Picture activity, for adolescents 171–172
co-change agent, parents as 25, 44, 49, 75
Cognitive Behavioral Play Therapy 23
cognitive development 22
Color by Number Picture activity, for adolescents 173–174
communication: deficits in 7; skills 10, 200; social interaction and 18; struggles 18–19
Communication Blocks activity, for adolescents 190–191
confidentiality 41–42
connection ability 14, 26
Cross, A. 22

Dawson, G. 19
Delloso, A. M. 17
Diagnostic and Statistical Manual of Mental Disorders, 5th Edition 7, 8–9
Dienstmann, R. 19
Divide and Conquer activity, for adolescents 80–81
Domino Challenge activity, for adolescents 123–124
Drewes, A. A. 25
dysregulation issues 11, 33–35, 183

Echterling, L. G. 32
emotional development 22
emotional regulation 6, 9, 14, 19, 26, 31, 70, 181
Emotional Story activity, for children 142–144
ethical considerations, in AutPlay therapy groups 40–42
executive functioning 11
eye gaze 12

family/parent involvement, in AutPlay groups 38–40; *see also* parents
fear of making mistakes 11
Feelings Collage activity, for adolescents 175–176
Filial Therapy 23, 37
Fill My Bucket activity, for children 126–127
Find the Prize activity, for children 130–131

Follow Me Approach (FMA), in AutPlay Therapy 27–28, 43–44, **44**, 49, 54
Follow the Leader activity, for adolescents 192–193

generalization, of social skills 10, 38
goodbye ritual: in AutPlay play and social skill groups 51, 77; in other languages 88–89
Grandin, T. 2
Grant, R. J. 13, 14, 23, 25
Group High Five activity, for adolescents 117–118
Group Machine activity, for children 163–164
Group Readiness Questionnaire 21
groups 43; assessing members 45–46, 71–72; children participation in 46, 72; ethical considerations for 40–42; generating interest in 45, 71; implementing play therapy interventions in 31; meetings 46–47, 48, 72–74, 74; organization of 45, 71; peer 17, 23, 198; play 10; size of 46, 72; types 3–4, 27, 28, 29–42; *see also* AutPlay® Therapy play groups; AutPlay® Therapy social skills groups

Hand Jive activity, for adolescents 178
Have You Filled A Bucket Today? (McCloud) 126
Higashida, N. 1
hyperarousal/hyperarousal 14

individualized education program (IEP) 7
informed consent and confidentiality 41–42
intellectual disability 8
interventions (social skills), for adolescents: *Act As If* activity 177; *Architects* activity 188–189; *Bubble Tag* activity 167–168; *Circle Picture* activity 171–172; *Color by Number Picture* activity 173–174; *Communication Blocks* activity 190–191; *Divide and Conquer* activity 80–81; *Domino Challenge* activity 123–124; *Feelings Collage* activity 175–176; *Follow the Leader* activity 192–193; *Group High Five* activity 117–118; *Hand*

Jive activity 178; *I Spy* activity 179–180; *Keep It Going* activity 169–170; *Magazine Minute* activity 196–197; *Make a Monster* activity 200–201; *Monster Collaborative Drawing* activity 103–104; *Oops and Ouch* activity 185–187; *Personal Space* activity 92–93; *Play-Doh Relax* activity 194–195; *Safe Zones* activity 183–184; *Secret Message* activity 128–129; *Symphony Composers* activity 98; *Topic Tower Builders* activity 108–109; *Wall Draw* activity 198–199; *What to Say Scripts* activity 181–182; *Where I Stand* activity 86–87; *Where it Belongs* activity 112–113
interventions (social skills), for children: *Animal Feelings* activity 155–156; *Animal Pairs* activity 136–137; *Backward Moves* activity 165–166; *Bingo Friends* activity 138–139; *Boatman* activity 147–148; *Bubbles Social Skills* activity 140–141; *Emotional Story* activity 142–144; *Fill My Bucket* activity 126–127; *Find the Prize* activity 130–131; *Group Machine* activity 163–164; *Listen and Speak* activity 84–85; *Midline Mirror Moves* activity 153–154; *Monster Maker* activity 101–102; *Move It! Move It!* Activity 116; *Progressive Balloon Game* activity 151–152; *Quiet and Loud* activity 78–79; *Roles and Turns* activity 134–135; *Safe and Unsafe* activity 149–150; *Scavenger Hunt* activity 121–122; *Space Mistakes* activity 132–133; *Space Please!* activity 90–91; *Sword Balloons* activity 159–160; *Symphony Composers* activity 96–97; *Together Balloons* activity 145–146; *Topic Tower Builders* activity 106–107; *Volcano* activity 157–158; *Where it Belongs* activity 111; *WRJMD* activity 161–162
introspection 12–13
I Spy activity, for adolescents 179–180

Jamison, T. R. 16
joint attention 12

Keep It Going activity, for adolescents 169–170
Koenig, K. 2, 16
Kottman, T. 30

Landreth, G. L. 36
language development 22
limit setting models: ACT 36–37; Adlerian Play Therapy 38; Filial Therapy 37; for managing disruptive behavior 35–38; practicing 48; three R's 35–36
Line Up game 88
Listen and Speak activity, for children 84–85
listening skills 77, 130
Luck, J. 18
Lyons, T. 6

MacDonald, J. 27
Magazine Minute activity, for adolescents 196–197
Make a Monster activity, for adolescents 200–201
McCloud, Carol 126
McPartland, J. 19
Midline Mirror Moves activity, for children 153–154
Milestones Autism Resources 13
Monster Collaborative Drawing activity, for adolescents 103–104
Monster Maker activity, for children 101–102
movement intervention, for children 116

Name Game 110
neurotypical vs. atypical play in children, guide for **24–25**

Oops and Ouch activity, for adolescents 185–187
Ozonoff, S. 19

Papaefstathiou, E. 16
parents: and child play time 51; as co-change agent 25, 44, 49, 75; conducting AutPlay interventions at home 26–27; handling unwanted behavior 49, 75; hosting meeting with group 47–48, **48**, 70–71, 73–74, **74**; incorporating into AutPlay groups 38–40; meeting place options for 47–48, **48**, 70–71, 73–74, **74**; participation in AutPlay play groups

46, 49, 72; practicing limit setting model 48; Session Overview Form for 51, 77; training component 26–27
participation opportunity, in AutPlay play and social skill groups: for parents 38–40, 46, 49, 72; to sharing anything with groups 76–77
partners in play, professionals as 30
peer/group play 10, 23
perseveration 12
Personal Space activity, for adolescents 92–93
physical removal 36
play: benefits in 22; challenges 22; change agents 25–26; development 47, 73; interventions 23, 26, 31; as learning tool 22; as modality to teaching social skills 31; neurotypical vs. atypical development **24–25**; skills 10, 14, 22–23, 70; and social time 50–51; therapeutic factors 22, 25–26; and therapeutic relationship 32; therapists 41
Play-Doh Relax activity, for adolescents 194–195
playful flow 32
play groups *see* AutPlay® Therapy play groups
play therapy: directive interventions 26, 31, 43, 70–71; groups 43; limit setting models in 35–38; theories 23; *see also* AutPlay® Therapy
Play Therapy Best Practices 41
pretend and imaginative play 10
problem solving 22, 26, 112, 121
processing speed 11
professionals 3–4, 11; in AutPlay Therapy groups 30; developing assessment procedure 14; engaging with child 27–28, 43, **44**; ethical considerations 40–42; in Follow Me Approach (FMA) 27–28, 43–44, **44**; handling unwanted behavior 33–35, 48–49, 74–75; implementing play therapy interventions in groups 31; limit setting models, use of 35–38, 48; as partners in play 30; providing psychoeducation to parents 40; roles of 30, **44**, 45, 71; transitions, following child 27, 43, **44**; *see also* 10-session guide; interventions (social skills), for adolescents; interventions (social skills), for children

Progressive Balloon Game activity, for children 151–152

Quiet and Loud activity, for children 78–79
Quinn, A. M. 17

receptive language 10, 14, 19
reciprocity 12, 19
redirection 35
reflective statements **44**, 52
regulation ability 11
relationships: development 7–8, 27, 32, 36, 40, 43; positive 18
removal 36
replacement 35–36
rigid (literal) thinking 10–11
Roles and Turns activity, for children 134–135

Safe and Unsafe activity, for children 149–150
Safe Zones activity, for adolescents 183–184
Scavenger Hunt activity, for children 121–122
Schaefer, C.E. 22, 25
school, individuals with ASD in 6–7, 14, 17
Schuttler. J. O. 16
Secret Message activity, for adolescents 128–129
self-advocacy 13
self-reflection (introspection) 12–13
sensory processing 13, 26
Session Overview Form 48, 51, 77
Siri, K. 6
social cognition 17
social competence 16
social functioning: AutPlay Therapy interventions to increasing 26, 31; deficits 11–12, 14–15, 16–17; issues 6; *see also* social skills
social interactions 17
social reciprocity 12
social rules, categories of 2
social skills 1–2, 16–21; categorization guide 19, **20**; children with ASD 13, 70; competence in 16; development 3, 15, 16, 47, 70, 73; generalization of 10, 38; play therapy interventions 26; scripts 140–141; training 17, 19; *see also* interventions (social skills), for adolescents; interventions (social skills), for children

social skills groups *see* AutPlay® Therapy social skills groups
social skills interventions 2–3, 4, 32–33, 38, 77; *see also* interventions (social skills), for adolescents; interventions (social skills), for children
Space Mistakes activity, for children 132–133
Space Please! activity, for children 90–91
splintered skill development 9
Stewart, A. L. 32
Stoika P. 27
structure: AutPlay play groups 45; AutPlay social skill groups 71
structured play 32
structuring statement 50
Sword Balloons activity, for children 159–160
Symphony Composers activity, for children and adolescents 96–98
Syriopoulou-Delli, C. K. 16

table, utilization in play group session 50
"That's Like Me" statement 82
theory of mind 12, 190
therapeutic factors of play 22, 25–26
therapeutic relationship development 32, 36
Theraplay® 23
three R's limit setting model 35–36
Together Balloons activity, for children 145–146
Topic Tower Builders activity: adolescent version 108–109; children version 106–107
tracking statements **44**, 52

uneven development 9–10

VanFleet, R. 37
Volcano activity, for children 157–158

Wall Draw activity, for adolescents 198–199
What to Say Scripts activity, for adolescents 181–182
Where I Stand activity, for adolescents 86–87
Where it Belongs activity: adolescent version 112–113; children version 111
writing and other academic skills 12
WRJMD (walk, run, jump, march, and dance) activity, for children 161–162

For Product Safety Concerns and Information please contact our EU
representative GPSR@taylorandfrancis.com Taylor & Francis Verlag GmbH,
Kaufingerstraße 24, 80331 München, Germany

Printed and bound by CPI Group (UK) Ltd, Croydon, CR0 4YY
08/06/2025
01897007-0005